Amish

Folk

Medicine

ALSO BY PATRICK QUILLIN, PH.D., R.D.

Adjuvant Nutriton in Cancer Treatment

Beating Cancer with Nutrition

Healing Nutrients

Healing Secrets from the Bible

The LaCosta Book of Nutrition

The LaCosta Prescription for Longer Life

Safe Eating

Patrick Quillin, Ph.D., R.D.

Amish

Folk

Medicine

Artwork by Noreen Quillin

Foreword by A. Gordon Reynolds, M.D.
Inspired by Sarah Weaver & Fani's Books

The Leader Company,Inc.,931 N.Main, N. Canton, OH 44720
ISBN 1-886898-01-4

Publisher's Cataloging in Publication Data
Quillin, Patrick.
Amish folk medicine: do Amish people know
something that doctors don't?/Patrick Quillin. p.   cm.

      1. Amish—medicine. 2. Alternative medicine.   I.
      Title
      R733.Q85 1995   615.5
Library of Congress No. 95-077115

Printed in the United States of America.
Page Design and Typography, Elizabeth Strauss

Produced & distributed by BookWorld Services, Inc.
1933 Whitfield Park Loop   Sarasota, FL 324243
24-hour order lines: 800/444-2524   *Fax:* 800/777-2525

Foreword

Nature has provided us with an extraordinary array of non-toxic therapeutic substances. When I began practicing medicine in the early 1950s, medical science was on the threshold of the most rapid advances in its history. My medicine bag expanded from a few antibiotics to include thousands of options for potent medicines. While teaching at the University of California Los Angeles, I found it challenging to keep up with the waves of information that swept through medical science.

Over three decades, I delivered more than 3500 babies in my private practice and noticed a dramatic change among the medical community. We gradually veered from watching the patient and using minimal intervention toward watching computer monitors and employing substantial medical intervention. Cesarean rates went from 4% to 35% in many hospitals from 1960 to 1990.

The upshot of all this "progress" was to lose a connection to our roots of folk medicine. I am still awestruck by our technical wizardry. Computer X rays (CAT scans) provide more information than we used to get from autopsies. Laser surgery brings a new level of accuracy even to the most gifted surgeon. An endless array of disease-specific drugs are available for nearly every symptom.

On the other hand, I am equally impressed with the apothecary that nature provides us in foods, herbs, and other low-risk approaches. As I became more convinced of the superior therapies offered by the body's own healing mechanisms, I switched from gynecology to preventive medicine and returned to school. My eight years as Medical Director of the world's largest health spa, at La Costa in southern California, proved to me that whenever available, nature's cure is the safest and most effective. Often, nature is the only option that really works.

We must not abandon all the progress that medical science has made. Yet, we must begin a vigorous campaign to incorporate the natural medicine that allowed us to survive this long—folk medicine. For most of the world, throughout most of history, the only medicine was folk medicine. Remedies are only passed on for multiple generations if they work.

I am impressed by the research Dr. Quillin has conducted to gather this book. My personal projection on the direction of the healing arts is that we will eventually weave together the best of modern science with the best of ancient natural cures. Together they will form a hybrid method of clinically effective and cost-effective means of treating diseases. This book represents a milestone in that pursuit. We can learn a great deal from our Amish brethren. I must stress that a healthy lifestyle—which includes proper exercise, good nutrition, and a positive attitude—will go a long way to prevent illness. Read this book and watch your health improve while your medical bills are reduced.

A. Gordon Reynolds, MD
co-author of
The La Costa Book of Nutrition
San Diego, California

Table of Contents

How to Use This Book

"Nature, to be commanded, must be obeyed."
—Francis Bacon 1620 A.D..

Why the Amish?

There must be a better way! . . . Too many people
have said that in my presence. Americans spend over
$800 billion annually on health care. And what do we
get for this unprecedented investment? We have
among the highest rates in the world for heart disease,
cancer, diabetes, osteoporosis, neonatal death, and
mental illness, as well as widespread chronically
annoying symptoms like depression, constipation,
and fatigue. So how do the Amish and other simple
people survive without the benefits of modern
medicine?

1

Why do we tolerate our health care system that the World Health Organization has called "invasive, controlling, and sometimes disabling." Where drugs can cost more than gold, ounce for ounce, with one arthritis medication costing 100 times that of gold ... where the side effects of many drugs can be more harmful than the condition itself ... where it has been proven that a life-threatening $30,000 open-heart by-

pass surgery does nothing to extend the life span of the average heart disease patient . . . where a Harvard professor has compiled impressive statistics to show that the 22-year $30 billion "War on Cancer" has been a dismal failure.[1]

This book project began as a quest to find the wisdom of the "old ones", people who live a simpler lifestyle, closer to Nature. A group of Americans that epitomize the simple life are the Amish people. Although human history is rich with texts on

2

folk medicine, much of it was ignored due to our enthusiasm for modern science. People who valued a simpler way of life—the Amish, Native Americans, Asians, and other groups—have preserved these natural remedies out of the need for survival.

The Amish movement was born in 1525 A.D. with the Anabaptist of Reformation times. Most of today's Amish are descendants of the followers of Jakob Ammann, a 17th century Mennonite leader who advocated strict community conformity. Today, about 70,000 Amish are dispersed in 50 or so communities in the United States and Canada. Through their simple and self-sufficient lifestyle and shunning modern conveniences, such as electricity and automobiles, they have become the American repositories of folk medicine.

While I began this project with a certain suspicion about the mysterious Amish who shun society, I concluded my research with a newfound respect for their work ethic, community spirit, family values, superior health, and low-stress life. Our current unwieldy health care system could learn much from the Amish. Shunning modern medicine and not willing to lie down and die, they tried an endless array of folk cures to relieve symptoms and oftentimes to save the lives of their children. The Amish, and other groups, have maintained that health and happiness are attainable only when humans are in harmony with the laws of God and Nature—not in trying to find loopholes to these laws, as modern man has done.

The Amish try to incorporate ancient Biblical recommendations into their everyday lifestyle: hard work, respect for each other's rights, kind treatment toward the less fortunate, friendliness, moderation, pleasures of family, and sincerity.

Hence, we need to credit these "backward" people, not only for their efforts at retaining our valuable heritage of natural healing, but also for their own enviable society at a time when the very fabric of mod-

4

ern society is fraying at the edges.

On a personal note, I was having chronic sinus problems for more than a year, in spite of trying many nutritional and medical approaches. With great skepticism, I tried one of the cures listed in this book. *Swab the inside of the nose with Vicks® (a poultice of camphor, menthol, a special grade spirits of turpentine, eucalyptus, cedar leaf oil, myristica, thymol).* It worked. I could breath again.

I had a suspicious skin spot on my face from years of excess exposure to the sun. While the reigning champion in modern medicine, Retin-A® salve, did nothing but irritate the spot, a poultice of herbs and zinc oxide (described in this book) completely healed the skin spots in 2 weeks.

I travel extensively. Sometimes I find myself in an uncomfortable or noisy hotel room at night with a big presentation to give in the morning and no chance for sleep. Sleeping pills would leave me feeling drugged the next day. Other folk remedies did not work. So I tried an Amish remedy—valerian root capsules (3 at bedtime)—and found no problem sleeping and no problem getting up the next morning.

For 17 years, my wife tried endless over-the-counter medical preparations to heal herself of two planters' warts on her feet. The method used by the Amish, castor oil salve, took the warts off in 2 weeks. My wife also found quick and easy relief for a urinary tract infection by taking cranberry extract pills, as described in this book. I now agree with Halfdan Mahler, MD, Director General of the World Health Organization, who tells us *The age-old arts of the herbalists must be tapped. Many of the plants familiar to the wise woman really do have the healing powers that tradition attaches to them.* My wife and I are believers.

Make no mistake about it, nature has an answer for most health ills. We did not develop modern medicine until the last 50 years. Which means that for 99.9% of our history, folk medicine must be credited for allowing us to survive this long. By 60 A.D., the Roman surgeon Dioscorides was the first to gather notes on the folk medicine cures of the various countries that he visited. It was not until the 15th century that this knowledge was returned by way of Arabs, who found and used Dioscorides book.[2] Today, the World Health Organization estimates 80% of the world's people rely entirely on folk medicine for healing.[3]

Scientifically Valid Herbal Medicine

Since the days of the Old Testament, humans have been tapping the enormous healing power of herbs. We see this in Genesis 1:12, *And the earth brought forth vegetable, and God saw that it was good.* and Genesis 1:29 *And God said, "Behold I have given you every herb bearing seed, that is upon the face of the earth."*

Multi-national, multi-billion dollar drug companies have not ignored the importance of herbs. One third of all prescription drugs sold in the United States are herbal extracts. Vincristine, a potent anticancer drug for childhood leukemia, is made from the periwinkle plant. Digitalis, a powerful drug for an ailing heart, is made from the foxglove plant.

Nearly 2,000 years ago, folk medicine guides recommended drinking a brew made from white willow leaves to treat gout. White willow contains naturally occurring aspirin, a favorite drug of today's pharmacists for analgesic purposes (pain killing).

A poultice made from bread mold has been recommended for centuries in the treatment of infections. Bread mold contains penicillin.

South American natives use darts dipped in their local herb curare to paralyze their prey. Curare is now a drug regularly used in modern hospitals as a muscle relaxant.

Spanish explorers found that tincture of cinchona bark from Brazilian forests could be used to treat malaria. Cinchona bark contains quinine, which has been the standard of malaria treatment for centuries. (As the rain forests of the world are being leveled at a rate of space the size of Pennsylvania each year, we are becoming painfully aware of the healing treasures that are lost forever from our clear-cut rain forests.)

Potency and Safety

Garlic is such a potent healing force that if it were not a food, it would take 10 years of scientific research and cost $5 million to fully test this "wonder drug" before the Food and Drug Administration would approve garlic for sale.

While there are some toxic plants, most of the folk cures listed in this book are far safer than the alternative prescription drug. For example, an extract of blueberries (drug name: *Pecarin*) is the preferred treatment for diarrhea in Swedish hospitals. An extract of cranberries is still the best method of treating female urinary tract infections. One of the primary drugs prescribed to lower cholesterol, *clofibrate*, has been shown in a

World Health Organization study to markedly increase the risk for cancer, liver disease, pancreas inflammation, and ironically, heart disease, which is it supposed to prevent.[4]

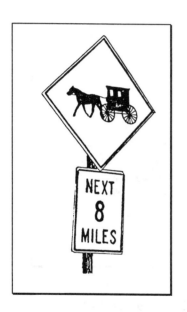

Meanwhile, the folk medicine treatment, which includes vitamin C, niacin, oat bran, chromium, and herbs, is far more effective and has no toxicity.

One of the ironic situations in American health care is that natural substances cannot be patented, hence companies have no financial motivation to develop natural products for health care.

Many companies spend millions of research dollars trying to create a synthetic derivative that will provide health benefits comparable to the already-proven natural compound. This tremendous effort is spent so that drug companies can patent the substance and reap much higher profits.

Improving on Mother Nature?

Folk medicine is heavily based on extracts from foods and herbs, which is the main limiting factor in folk medicine—unreliable concentrations of the active ingredient. No two pieces of wood are alike in grain. No two samples of cow liver are identical in nutrient content. And no two pieces of garlic have equal concentrations of *allicin*, the active ingredient. Over 2000 years ago, Queen Cleopatra of Egypt used fresh cut aloe vera leaves to soothe burns. Unfortunately, not everyone has access to fresh aloe plants, which encouraged many people to try concentrating the active ingredient in aloe. However, not until recently have chemists been able to isolate and concentrate the fragile molecule from aloe to achieve more predictable results in health care.

Until recently, folk medicine was somewhat of a hit or miss approach, which worked on some occasions and not on others. The herbalist was unsure of the quality and quantity of active ingredients in the plants used. Lacking sensitive lab equipment that we now have to test these active ingredients, folk healers ascribed their unpredictable results to fate or the inborn talent of the healer. We now have the opportunity to join the best of modern science and folk medicine by using herbal extracts standardized for potency, which yield far more predictable health results.

That is why some of the recommendations in this book provide for more exacting ways of getting the healing results that you need. Rather than relying on your ability to harvest and process fresh ginseng to protect the delicate active ingredients, you can buy it in pill form at any time from reputable mail-order companies.

Following each symptom is a list of original Amish folk cures. For some symptoms, there is an additional section, called *Other*, which highlights equally valuable folk and scientific information that may help the reader. This book is not intended to be an all-encompassing collection of natural-healing approaches. It is intended to provide the Amish folk remedies plus a few other non-toxic approaches.

No Vested Interests

Most recommendations in this book refer to a generic product, such as red clover tops, vinegar, or ginseng; rather than to a specific company or product name. A selection of vendors is listed in the back of the book which includes quality mail-order firms where remedies listed in this book can be purchased. Please be assured that I have no vested interest in selling these products. The vendors are listed for your benefit, not my benefit or that of the companies listed.

Many Other Possible Therapies

This book approaches healing from the standpoint of foods, herbs, and other natural home remedies that are used by the Amish and other cultures who shun modern medicine. Using the methods in this book, you should need no assistance.

Beyond this book, there is an extensive array of alternative-health approaches, including acupuncture, homeopathy, reflexology, schools of psychological therapy, color therapy, aroma therapy, and more. Usually treatment in these fields requires someone trained in that field to assist you. Check the Appendix for a bibliography of textbooks that offer information on natural therapies.

Healthy Lifestyle

One expert stated, "We are digging our graves with our teeth." A Harvard University Framingham study said: "Our way of life is linked to our way of death." Heart disease, cancer, arthritis, diabetes, osteoporosis and decades of nagging symptoms are diverse manifestations of the same unhealthy lifestyle.

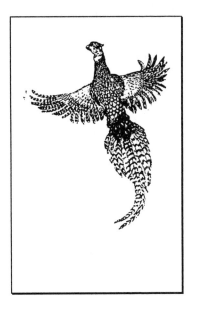

Each person's symptom merely expresses the weakest link in the chain of his or her body. The Amish live a generally healthy lifestyle—no liquor or tobacco, moderation in fresh unprocessed food intake, and plenty of exercise and fresh air.

In order to make this book a valuable lifetime guide, I have included in the Appendix a general description of a healthy lifestyle. Realize that, if you are living the typical unhealthy American lifestyle, all of the herbs in the world cannot overcome a destructive way of life. For this book to have a powerful impact on your health, I encourage you to read the Appendix on healthy lifestyle and to incorporate those recommendations along with the remedies in this book. That is how the Amish benefit most from these folk cures.

As a by-product of their atypical lifestyle, the Amish have far more treatments for bee stings and minor problems of pregnancy than for alcoholism and insomnia. While the Amish are people of a simple lifestyle, they are not simple minded. Modern society has favored the "magic bullet" pill approach to healing—keep living the way you are; just take a pill and all symptoms and disease will magically disappear. More realistic in their approach, the Amish have categorized and use the many forces that make up good health.

THE FORCES COMPRISING GOOD HEALTH   1 Solar Therapy

In Genesis, God said *Let there be light.* Without light there is no life. The food chain of life begins with the sun's action on green plants. Animals eat plants. Humans are omnivorous (*omni=everything*) and therefore, eat some plants and animals. Everything we consume comes directly or indirectly from the sun.

Most creatures and all humans are heavily dependent on both light and color for health. Scientists have discovered a common condition called Seasonal Affective Disorder, or SAD, which leaves people feeling depressed throughout the dark winter months. The cure is full-spectrum lights, which can be purchased. The cause is a brain response. The brain has a meter (pineal gland) that measures the quality and quantity of light going into our eyes. Without adequate light, many people get depressed. Surrounding colors are also important—green is healing; pink is relaxing; red is energizing; and so on.

Humans are designed to eat fresh foods. The Amish tell us that much of the "light energy" is lost from processing foods. Chemical fertilizers and highly-refined junk food do not have this crucial light energy.

The Amish people work outside as much as possible to further emphasize the importance of light. As much as possible, the Amish eat from their own vegetable gardens. They constantly tend kitchen gardens of sprouts. Scientists have found that sprouted seeds improve in biological value of protein, enzyme, and vitamin content by up to 600%.

To sprout seeds into young plants, get untreated seeds of alfalfa, mung beans, sunflower, lentils, radish, wheat grass, rye, corn, rice, peas, and millet. Soak them overnight in a glass jar. Rinse them 3-5 times daily. Let stand inverted with a screen cover to keep the sprouts in and allow the water to drain out.

To obtain more light-energy food, toss organically grown fruits and vegetables (or peeled commercial produce) into a high-speed blender to make juice. Drink a glass of this juice daily. Steep the crushed leaves of your favorite herb (mint works well) in a gallon glass jar in the sun to make herb tea.

The body also can be-
come ill from looking
through the wrong color
tinted lenses. Wear
sunglasses tinted blue or
green.

Use full spectrum light
bulbs in your home or get plenty of outdoor natural
light. Wear a hat in the sun. Do not get too much sun
on the skin. Scientists have found that a combination
of poor diet (not enough antioxidants) coupled with
too much sun has led to an epidemic of skin cancer
and cataracts in America.

Clay, mud, and spring water all form an important
part of Amish healing traditions. Immersion in mud
baths, volcanic mud, hot spring waters, and the wet
sand by the seashore can be instrumental in purging
the body of toxins. Clay masques are used to purify
facial pores. Clay poultices can relieve sore eye lids.
Kao lin (Chinese clay) taken internally helps purge

the intestines of toxins and relieve diarrhea. This same clay is sold as the product Kaopectate®.

When using clay and mud from the earth, be sure to eliminate the possibility that animal excrement with its accompanying parasitic worms are present. A great health risk for both city and farm dwellers is parasites. The Amish regularly take male fern root and garlic to purge the body of parasites.

Foods that are particularly rich in light energy in-

clude: sprouts, fish liver oils, liver, eggs, yeast, and fresh green and orange fruits and vegetables. The Amish consume large amounts of fresh fruit in the winter, in addition to their red clover tea. Winter is the time that many people fall into a scurvy-like condition due to lack of vitamin C—but not if you follow the guidelines of the Amish and consume many light-energy foods.

21

Many of these fresh wild-grown herbs are rich sources of minerals—lamb's quarters and okra pods provide calcium; watercress provides sulphur, dandelion and stinging nettle for iron; kelp (seaweed) provides iodine; mullein leaves provide magnesium; garlic provides sulphur and selenium; grape juice provides potassium; oat straw provides silicon; and more.

The Amish slowly chew root of ginseng all day. There is an abundance of scientific evidence showing the rejuvenating properties of ginseng. Not until modern chemists could isolate the active ingredient in ginseng, ginsenosides, could they conduct research to determine its amazing therapeutic value.

In hundreds of studies well outlined in Dr. Michael Murray's book, *The Encyclopedia of Natural Medicine,* ginseng has proven to be an adaptogen, a substance that allows the body to better tolerate physical and mental stress; improves blood glucose regulation to help diabetics; elevates sexual function in men and women; inhibits tumor growth; stimulates the immune system; stabilizes blood pressure (raises or lowers, whichever is needed); lowers fats in the blood; increases the liver's ability to detoxify; and more.

2 Herbal Therapy

The world's greatest pharmacy lies in the humble parts of plants scattered throughout the planet. While there are dangerous chemicals in some plants (See the Appendix for poisonous plants), the therapeutic benefits of herbal extracts prove that we must pursue this avenue of healing; but with caution and attention to the wisdom of the old ones who have learned through experience.

23

3 Physiotherapy

The muscles, bones, and circulatory system are maintained by following a set of health laws. When these tissues suffer, so does the rest of the body. Exercise and body maintenance are crucial. Eating foods that nourish these valuable tissues is also important.

4 Diet Therapy

Maintaining proper digestion, elimination, absorption, and periodic fasting is crucial for health.

5 Respiratory Therapy

Jesus compared the Holy Spirit to the wind, blowing invisibly yet influencing us quite visibly. In James 4:14, we read, *What is your life? It is even a vapor, that appears for a little time, and then vanishes away.*

Pneuma refers to both breath and spirit. Before modern medicine, people used a mirror under the sinuses to determine death, measuring the absence of breath. Since the yogis of India 5000 years ago, we have known that air is the most crucial of all nutrients. We can survive weeks without food and days without water, but only a few minutes without air. Maintaining the health of the body parts that inhale and filter air is important. While polluted air is defined as more than 2,000 particles in a section of air half the size of a sugar cube, many cities average 15,000 particles of pollutants in that space of air on any given day.

The true paradox of life is that we require oxygen in all cells at all times to live. Yet the greatest destructive force in our body is oxygen. Oxygen allows us to extract 20 times more energy from food than anaerobic (without oxygen) bacteria. Yet oxygen also causes other molecules to rust, to oxidize, changing their structure. Just as iron outside your house is permanently ruined by oxygen, your body cells also can be affected. The secret answer to this paradox is antioxidants.

Antioxidants are vitamins (such as C, A, E), minerals (such as selenium), amino acids (such as cysteine), and other components (such as Coenzyme Q-10) which allow oxygen to be a friend and not a sabboteur within your body. Breathe properly and you live. Rust inside and you will suffer and die prematurely from the corrosive effects of oxygen. Breathe properly and take optimal amounts of antioxidants and you will get all of the benefits of oxygen without the toxic side effects. The Amish people have practiced this "best of both worlds" therapy since long before modern chemists understood the principle.

Full oxygenation of your body begins with proper deep breathing. Lie on your back on the floor with a book on your stomach. Begin inhaling by pushing the book up as high as possible with your stomach. Then finish filling your lungs by expanding your chest. This is proper breathing technique, which can be conducted while sitting, standing, or walking. It is important to first fill the diaphragm (lower lungs) with air. This allows oxygen to reach the tiny air sacs that bring oxygen from the lungs through the bloodstream to the cells.

It also is important to breathe clean air. Dust, pollen, mold, pollutants, and other air particulates can create hazards to your health. The Amish make sure that homes, basements, and attics are well ventilated. Homes should be cleaned regularly to avoid the buildup of dust and mold. The Amish use vaporizers, inhalers, and aromatic herbs to improve breathing. Remember, the breath of life is crucial.

6 Hydrotherapy

Two thirds of Earth's surface is covered with water. Two thirds of the weight of an adult is water. The ancient Greeks used to categorize all of life into the four elements of water, air, fire, and earth. Water is truly the river of life in our bodies. The Amish try to build their homes near running water to capture its energy and to reap the benefits of the calming sounds. Taking in and eliminating proper quantity and quality of water is critical for health.

Water is extremely valuable both inside and outside of the body. As a diaphoretic, a hot bath will induce sweating. Lukewarm water can induce vomiting. Warm water can help stimulate bowel movements. Bathing the brow during a fever helps to cool the body. Water is the primary cleansing agent we use to keep our homes and clothes clean. Water is equally crucial for cleansing our insides. Water dilutes the toxins in the body and encourages their elimination through the kidneys and sweat.

The early healing temples were all centered around water. From hot springs, to Scandinavian cold plunges, to seashore sand baths, to mud baths, humans have reveled in the healing properties of water.

7 Spiritual Therapy

The mind is the master organ. Hope, love, peace, and forgiveness are the springboards of good health; while hate, low self-esteem, and other negative emotions can cripple even the otherwise healthiest of individuals. The Amish have tried-and-proven methods for dealing with the emotional illness that can cause physical illness.

Love. God is love and love is what heals all. This law is first in Amish life.

Adversity. With a solid community of like-minded individuals, the Amish do not have insurance, because they have a support network of friends and family to care for them during troubled times. Interestingly enough, scientists now find that the greatest risk factor toward heart disease is loneliness.

Alms. Give away a portion of your wealth without boasting and you will be amply rewarded.

Anger. A soft answer turns away wrath (Prov. 15:1). Don't let the sun go down on your anger (Eph. 4:26). Settle quarrels quickly. Resentment will eat a person up like cancer. Forgive others so that you may be forgiven (Matthew 6:12).

Blessings. Count your blessings. Consider the generosity of the sun, wind, rain, and earth.

Curses. Overcome evil with good by blessing those who curse you. If your enemy is hungry, feed him and melt his fury with gentleness (Romans 12:20). Cursing and swearing are sure signs of a poor vocabulary.

Conscience. A clear conscience is the best pillow.

Contentment. He that is content has enough. The greatest wealth is to live content with little, for there is never want where the mind is satisfied.

Death. The Amish have simple unpretentious funerals, which manifest their philosophy: "Show me love while I am living, instead of trying to convince the undertaker."

Depression. Everyone will at some time face the feelings of depression and defeat. The best prescription for depression is to count your blessings. Amish women recognize the possibility of post-partum (after pregnancy) depression and take extra B-vitamins and red clover top liquid extract to counter this condition.

Envy. A person who is content with his or her lifestyle is not easily moved by high-pressure advertising about what you need to feel fulfilled. It is not so much what you eat that makes you sick, but what is eating you because of what you are looking at and wanting.

Family. Close-knit families are the rule, instead of a generation gap and disrespect for older people. Grand-parents are not warehoused in institutions, but kept at home in their own cottage on the farm (called the *Dawdy Haus*). Due to their community support net, the Amish can shun society security, welfare, government hand-outs, and crop insurance.

Fear. There is no fear in love, but perfect love cast out fear. (1 John 4:18)

Happiness. Happiness is a healthy outlook on life. If you cannot change your circumstances, then you can change yourself to adapt to those circumstances. Happiness is found by avoiding pride, anger, malice, lust, greed, fashion, and vanity.

Holidays. The Amish cherish their holidays and do only the most basic chores for their animals on these special occasions. Always honor the Sabbath with rest and praise.

Humor. Laughing exercises the lungs, heart, and adrenal glands while stimulating the mind to produce endorphins, which give us both pleasure and good health. Laughter relieves tension and fear.

Modesty. Outward plainness allows inward beauty to develop, otherwise one acts a part with cosmetics and costumes. *Whose adorning let it not be that outward adorning of plaiting the hair, and of wearing of gold, or of putting on of apparel; but let it be the hidden man of the heart, in that which is not corruptible, even the ornament of a meek and quiet spirit, which is in the sign of God of great price.* (1 Peter 3:3)

Simplicity. Do not become slaves to machines, materialism, and greed. Avoid outside clutter and baubles, so that a person can concentrate on the true meaning of life, which is to praise God, develop his or her own talents, help others, and to rejoice in being.

Thanksgiving. It is hard to find a thankful person who is also unhappy. Replace criticism, complaining, and accusations with praise, thanksgiving, and encouragement.

Touch. In one old Amish practice, members greet other members with a kiss as a sign of family closeness. The Amish enjoy regular massages of the feet, scalp, and back. Massage relieves tension. "If you want to keep your ticker ticking, then don't wind it too tight." Certain Amish dedicate their careers to the ministry of healing touch. Touching is important for human health.

Work ethic. Parents want their children to be hard workers, producing useful fruits of labor, not lazy parasites trying to live by their wits while loafing. Industrious children become industrious adults.

Parting Comments of Caution

Your health is important and sometimes fragile. If you have nagging symptoms, see your doctor. Bring this book to your doctor and work together as a team. Your doctor wants you to get well. I want you to have the best of health and not delay in receiving proper treatment when the symptoms warrant further attention.

We have a tendency to develop stereotypes. One such is "everything that is synthetic is bad for you and everything that is natural is good for you." There are many noteworthy exceptions to that oversimplification, including hemlock, the venom of the Black Widow spiders, and botulism extract from food poisoning. Many plants are harmful. Some are even lethal. Mushrooms are so difficult to distinguish between the good and the bad, that even experts are extremely cautious about foraging for wild mushrooms.

Nature's pharmacy is generous and under-utilized. Nature also contains some poisonous products that will harm the unwary. May you use good judgment and reap the abundant benefits found in this book.

Acne

Acne is caused by plugged up skin pores that grow infected with bacteria. Hence, excess oil secretions, dying skin tissue, excess bacteria, a crippled immune system, poor hygiene, poor diet, and hormonal imbalances associated with teen years and the menstrual cycle can bring on acne. Acne is most common in males ages 12 to 19 and females just before onset of their period. But acne is not something you must just accept.

- After washing the face in the evening, make a poultice of white sugar with a small amount of water and dab on the affected skin parts. Sugar has demonstrated anti-bacterial action.

- Take 1 tsp. sulphur and 2 tsp. baking molasses once or twice daily to cleanse the blood. Skin eruptions may increase initially. Continue therapy. The skin eruptions are an indication of cleansing the blood.

- Foods and supplements high in iodine can cause acne flare-ups. Avoid seafood, liver, cheese, and iodized salt for a while.

- Hot steam baths help reduce the viscosity of blackheads, which can then be scrubbed off or squeezed out. Do not squeeze pimples or whiteheads.

- Herbs that have reputed value in treating acne include: (best) burdock, chickweed, chlorophyll, dandelion, red clover, white oak bark, yellow dock, (good) aloe vera, cayenne, echinacea, ginseng, redmond clay sarsaparilla, and valerian. Take internally as a tea, or use as an external scrub.

- Take 3 tablets of activated charcoal 3 times daily.

- Consume an herbal combination of equal parts dandelion root, sarsaparilla root, burdock root, licorice root, echinacea, yellow dock root, kelp, cayenne, and chaparral.

- Take extra vitamin B-complex supplements.

- Ultraviolet radiation, from either the sun or a sunlamp, can kill facial bacteria while also drying up excess oil. Try getting a little sun to help acne.

- Some people get acne as a reaction to food. Chocolate is a primary inducer of acne. Try going without chocolate, tea, coffee, and colas.

- Diet has a major influence on acne. Eat less fat, more vegetables. For centuries, animal lovers have known that the quality of diet will be reflected in the animal's skin and coat. The same is true for humans.

Other:

- Hygiene and cleanliness are crucial. Wash your face with soap and warm water at least once daily. There are plenty of disinfectant lotions promoted as acne treatments. Those with benzoyl peroxide may help.

- Teen years are fraught with stress and intense emotions as children blossom into adults. Teens often develop nervous ticks, such as touching their hands to their face. The hands produce an acid in the sweat which can create skin infections. Keep your hands away from your face. You might notice how some people get acne only where their hands constantly stroke their face.

- Minimize use of make-up or do some investigative work to determine which type of make-up may contribute to flare-ups.

- Birth control pills can cause acne. Try another type of birth control pill or different method of birth control altogether.

- Oregon grape (Mahonia aquifolium) has been used successfully to treat acne. It has demonstrated properties as an antibiotic, anti-infective, and immune stimulant.[5] Dosages (all taken 3 times daily) include: tea from dried root (2–4 grams), tincture (6–12 ml or 1.5–3 tsp.), fluid extract (1–2 ml or 0.25–0.5 tsp.), and solid powder of 8–12% alkaloid content (250–500 mg).

Fats. While 60% of the fats consumed in America are hydrogenated (highly processed), studies have shown that animals fed a diet of 10% hydrogenated fats (a typical American diet) developed a deficiency of the essential fatty acid, linoleic acid.[6] Other researchers have found that acne sufferers often have a deficiency of linoleic acid in their skin region.[7]

- Recommendations: Eat less fat. Eat much less animal fat including cheese and ice cream. Eat no hydrogenated fat. Use olive oil for cooking and salad dressing. Consume 3 capsules or 1 T. daily of fish oil.

Zinc. Among the demands made on the body during teenage maturation is an increased need for zinc to provide for growth and sexual maturity. The typical teen diet is high in junk food which lacks zinc. Dr. Schachner found that a topical solution of zinc with the antibiotic erythromycin was very effective at healing acne.[8] Oral zinc supplements also healed acne.[9] In a particularly impressive experiment, 58% of acne subjects taking oral zinc supplements showed marked improvement in their condition, while the placebo group showed no improvement.[10]

- Recommendation: Take 50–100 mg/day of zinc

picolinate (a very well absorbed form of zinc).

Vitamin A works in many body systems and helps maintain the health of the skin. Research has shown that high doses of vitamin A improve acne.[11]

- Recommendations: Eat 3 oz. of liver at least once each week plus more green and orange fruits and vegetables, which are rich in the beta-carotene form of vitamin A. Take 25,000 iu of beta-carotene and 5,000 iu of vitamin A daily as pill supplements.

Chromium is an essential mineral involved in the processing of sugar in the bloodstream. Chromium from brewer's yeast was scientifically proven to treat acne in 9 human subjects.[12]

- Recommendation: Take 400 mcg/day of chromium as chromium picolinate, which is very absorbable, or 2 tsp. of high chromium yeast.

Vitamin E and Selenium. These two essential nutrients work in conjunction to create an important protective enzyme in the body called glutathione peroxidase. Six weeks of therapy with 400 mcg of selenium and 30 iu of vitamin E helped the majority of the 29 acne patients in this study.[13]

Age Spots

As we age, the processes of living take their toll and accumulate cellular debris, often called age spots. In some people, the liver is so undernourished or overwhelmed with toxins that it cannot excrete these waste products. Or lack of antioxidants to slow the "rusting" process of aging causes buildup of age spots. Life is basically an endless series of "bringing in the groceries," that is eating the right nutrients to feed the cells, and "taking out the trash" or excreting the waste products that are a natural by-product of living. If your body is not bringing in the right groceries or efficiently taking out the trash, then age spots occur.

- Herbs that may help include: dandelion, ginseng, gotu kola, licorice sarsaparilla.

Other:

Bilberry (Vaccinium myrtillus) has been shown to slow many of the processes of aging, act as an antioxidant, stabilize connection tissue (collagen), strengthen and stabilize blood vessels, and improve other side effects of aging.

- Recommendations: Take 4–8 oz. of fresh berries daily, or take 80–160 mg bilberry extract at 25% anthocyanidin, or 20–40 mg anthocyanosides daily.

Aging is a normal function of living. Premature aging is an accumulation of decades of neglect or abuse. Oxidation encourages the early destruction of tissue that leads to cataracts, blocked vessels, nonfunctioning minds, and cancer.

Recommendation: Use the overall healthy lifestyle and daily intake of antioxidants as described in the Appendix.[14]

Alcoholism

- Abstinence is the best method for prevention of the problem.
- Swallow 1 T. pure olive oil before drinking to relieve the craving for alcohol.

Other:

There is substantial evidence that amino acids, the building blocks that make up proteins, can provide relief from the craving for alcohol.

- Recommendations: Take 5 grams of L-glutamine daily, 2 grams of L-tryptophan, 3–4 grams of gamma-hydroxybutyric acid, 2 grams fish and borage oil emulsion (eicosapentaenoic acid plus gamma-linolenic acid) from BioSyn, 1 gram pantethine. Avoid sugar and caffeine to help stabilize blood sugar levels.[15]

One of the most productive nutrition scientists of the 20th century was Dr. Roger Williams of the University of Texas. Dr. Williams gathered data into a book showing that alcoholism can be a manifestation of unmet nutrient requirements. The complexities of the human body and its diet provide for no "magic bullet" nutrients, but rather require a total approach to satis-fying the biochemical needs of the body. Dr. Williams' book is highly recommended[16] and closely corresponds with the Appendix section on *Healthy Lifestyle.*

Allergies

- Chew honeycomb honey to help dry runny nose and unblock congested sinuses.
- Cleanse the sinuses with warm salt water. Prepare a solution using ½ tsp. salt (preferably sea salt) mixed in 8 oz. of filtered warm water. Bend over the sink and slowly in-hale through the nose, drawing the salt water solution into the sinuses. Plug your nose with your fingers to allow the solution to soak inside the si-nuses. Breathe through the mouth and hold water in sinuses for about 20 seconds. Expel

the solution along with any mucous and debris. Continue this process until the sinuses have been cleansed. This techniques proves a saving ritual for people who work around dust and sawdust. It helps to reduce time suffered with a cold. Also, this technique is helpful for bad breath and allergies.

Other:

- Tape or tie a small amount of food, dust, or whatever you think may be causing your allergy to your skin and leave it for 24 hours. If a red spot or rash appears, then you are probably allergic to that substance.
- Allergies can be caused by tension, emotion, toxic burden, or undigested protein particles.

Your body's allergic reactions are an overresponse of the immune system. One way to help subdue the symptoms of an allergy is to take vitamin C to suppress the release of histamines.

- Recommendations: Start by taking 2 grams/day of ascorbic acid. Then add 1 additional gram each day until you are taking 12 grams/day. (Use 2 grams or less for children under 5 years.) Use a buffered form of vitamin C if digestive problems develop. The easiest and cheapest way to increase vitamin C intake is by using powdered form. Take 1 tsp. (contains 4 grams) mixed in a small glass of fruit juice, 3 times daily (total = 12 grams). Follow the guidelines for healthy lifestyle in the Appendix.

- Allergies can be caused by incomplete digestion of proteins, by low thyroid output, or by stress, calcium/magnesium deficiency, etc.[17] Take 3 digestive enzyme tablets at each meal for digestion of proteins. Take thyroid replacement medication for low thyroid and reduce or avoid stressors.

Appendicitis

The appendix is a small finger-like projection from the intestines which is an active part of digestion in rabbits and other herbivores, but is inactive in humans. This little side spur detour can accumulate debris which can become inflammed and infected. A burst appendix can be lethal, since the bacteria spills into the abdominal cavity and bloodstream. Seek medical attention promptly if you think the appendix is inflamed.

- One tsp. of flaxseed daily may prevent the problem.
- One tsp. of olive oil daily may prevent the problem.
- Roughage in the diet may prevent the problem.

Other

- People on low fiber diets are more likely to develop appendicitis.

Asthma

Asthma involves a reduction in the flow of air to the lungs. The bronchial tubes leading to the lungs can be constricted or inflammed, giving the person the feeling of suffocating.

- Avoid dusty, smoky, dirty air environments, especially for children.
- Drink tea from Breathe Easy tea brand, found in health food stores.
- Formulate a syrup from comfrey root, mullein, garlic, fennel seed, and lobelia in vegetable glycerine and apple cider vinegar.
- Take 4 T. aloe vera gel before meals and at bedtime (4 times daily) for 2 weeks.
- To relieve an asthma attack, steep 4 oz. powdered lobelia in 1 quart rum. Let stand for 1 week. Then strain. Take ½ tsp. of this solution during an attack or use 3 drops 3 times daily as a preventive measure.
- Many asthma attacks are incited by food allergies. Eliminate all highly-refined foods, such as sugar, white flour, homogenized

whole milk, coffee, black tea, soda, and chocolate.

- Take 3 capsules of equal parts marshmallow, mullein, comfrey, lobelia, and chickweed 3 times daily.
- For deep bronchial coughs, chew on peeled ginseng root.
- Take 10 drops of elderberry tincture 3 times daily to help coughs.
- Mix the following herbal ingredients: 3 parts coughwart, 3 parts sage, 3 parts plantain, 1 part mullein. Add 1 c. boiling water to the mix. Cool and strain. Take one tsp. of this fluid every hour.
- Mullein leaf (Aaron's rod) tea may be helpful.
- To relieve the suffocating feeling, press a very cold, wet rag against the forehead.

Other

- Food allergies are often the cause of asthma.[18]

- Food additives, such as metabisulfite or monosodium glutamate, can cause asthma.[19]
- Vitamin B-6 supplements (50–100 mg/day) have been shown to reduce the incidence and severity of childhood asthma attacks.[20]
- Vitamin C supplements (1–2 grams/day) can reduce asthma attacks by lowering the sensitivity of the asthmatic person.[21]
- Magnesium supplements (400–800 mg/day) have reduced the severity of asthma attacks in human subjects.[22]

Athlete's Foot (Foot Fungus)

This common condition is basically a fungal infection that thrives on warm, moist, dark places, such as the places between toes. Among the simple ways of making life tough on this fungus is to change the pH (acid/base balance) by soaking the feet in a solution of mild acid (like vinegar) or alkaline (like baking soda).

- Add ½ c. of vinegar to a bowl of very warm water and soak feet. Repeat daily.

- Apply undesine ointment, which is available wherever herbs and natural remedies are sold.

- Sprinkle baking soda in the bottom of shoes, on the feet, and in socks. Repeat daily. Baking soda is also helpful for sweaty and/or smelly feet.

- Apply the raw juice from jewelweed (touch-me-not).

- Apply a salve of lard, iodine, powdered eggshells, and sulphur.

- Wash feet often in a mild solution of boric acid.
- Rinse feet in tea made from jewelweed, nasturtium, and muskmelon.

Other

- Daily supplements of garlic (6–8 capsules) and Lactobacillus pills or yogurt will bolster the immune system to ward off this fungal infection.[23]

Bad Breath

Bad breath usually stems from either the sinuses or the stomach. If your sinuses are plugged, irritated, or infected, see the section on Allergies.

- Chew anise seeds after meals.
- Pare off root bark of sweet calamus. Then chew the bark meat inside.
- Take 5 grams daily of purified charcoal tablets to cleanse the stomach and intestines.

- Stomach problems can be caused by a multitude of lifestyle factors—stress, liquor, overeating, high fat meals, insufficient supply of digestive enzymes, and so on.
- Eat less fat and sugar and consume more green vegetables, such as spinach, kale, collards, beet greens, and broccoli.
- Peppermint tea helps a sour stomach.
- An herbal concoction, called *Digest Herbal*, composed of peppermint, Gentian root, goldenseal root, atractylodes root, dandelion root, licorice root, anise seed, burdock root, ginger root, and fennel seed is available from Zand Formulas.

Other

- For indigestion, avoid foods high in fat, spices, and milk curd, such as pizza. Take 2–4 tablets of digestive enzymes with each meal. Take 1–2 grams dried rhizome & roots of the herb, Gentian Lutea. Take one 10 grain hydrochloric acid tablet per meal. (Build up to a warm feeling in the stomach, then cut back). Eat more kiwi, papaya, and pineapple—all contain digestive enzymes.[24]

Baldness

(See Hair and Skin Care)

Bath (Hydrotherapy)

- Take a relaxing bath with the following herbs added: rose petals, mint leaves, sweet marjoram, lemon balm, verbena, and lavender.
- For healthy detoxification, add 1 c. Epsom salts to a hot bath and soak for 15 minutes.
- For aching muscles, add 2 T. dry mustard powder to hot bath and soak for 15 minutes.
- To help eliminate perspiration odors, add ½ c. bicarbonate of soda to hot bath.

Bedsores

People who are confined to bed for long periods
of time have a tendency to develop sores, pimples, open wounds, and other signs of skin
breakdown. Much of these problems are due to
poor circulation.

- Mix white sugar with an unbeaten egg
  white and apply the mixture to sores.
- Mix 1 tsp. white sugar with milk of magne-
  sia and hydrogen peroxide to form a poultice. Apply to sores and cover with bandage.
- Soak towels in warm Epsom salts and lay
  on sores. Once towels cool, apply a poultice
  plaster of clay pine.
- Make a salve from ½ oz. oil of wintergreen,
  1 oz. glycerine, 2 oz. of rubbing alcohol, 2 oz.
  water.
- Omit food high in fat, sugar, and salt from
  the diet to improve the comfort of the patient.
- Apply Preparation H® to sores.

Other:

- On the bed, use a variable firmness mattress, or a foam mattress topper, such as sheepskin, that encourages better circulation in the skin.
- Move or roll over as much as possible. Lying in one position for long periods of time nearly guarantees bedsores.

Bedwetting

Most people have the autonomic nervous and muscular development to keep the bladder muscles tight while they sleep. Bedwetters often outgrow this symptom as they mature. Yet many methods show that bedwetting after age 3 or 4 is easily treated.

- Bedwetting is often caused by deep sleeping. Set an alarm clock for the bedwetter to get up every 3 hours to urinate.
- Give the person 1–2 tsp. of honey before retiring.
- Avoid intake of fluids after 5 PM.
- Drink a solution of 1 tsp. Epsom salts dissolved in
  8 oz. water with each noon meal.
- Eat dandelion plant and root. The roots can be cut up and roasted for a coffee substitute.

Other:

- Bedwetting is another symptom of allergies[25]. By finding the offending food, the bedwetting often stops. Mostly likely food suspects include: milk and other dairy products, wheat, and beef. Refer to *Healing Nutrients* (Random House, 1987—see bibliography) for the chapter on isolating food allergies.

Bleeding

The clotting ability of our blood depends on a number of factors that influence "prostaglandin" production. Prostaglandins are extremely potent substances in the body which regulate everything from muscle contractions, to immune activity, to the clotting ability of the blood supply. Of course, excessive bleeding can be fatal and requires medical attention.

- Use tincture of boiled clover blossoms to bath fresh wounds and sores.
- If someone has just stepped on a nail or pitchfork, soak the foot in a bucket of warm water to which a handful of wood ashes has been added. Make sure that the injured

person has had a tetanus shot within the last 2 years.

- Soak fresh wounds that have closed in saffron tea for rapid healing.
- Apply a poultice of grated onion to a fresh wound or cut.
- Wash off bleeding sores with pure vinegar to help the blood coagulate.
- Apply powdered alum to cuts to cause the skin to close.
- Cover the cut with paper from an unglazed brown bag that has been wet with vinegar.
- Apply powdered cayenne pepper to the wound.
- Clean the wound with hydrogen peroxide before trying to close the wound.

Other:

- Vitamin K deficiency can cause excess bleeding. Best sources of vitamin K are eating green and orange vegetables or liver, and stimulating the growth of healthy intestinal bacteria by eating yogurt.[26]

- Poor clotting can be cause by excess consumption of aspirin, fish oil, or the use of
anticoagulant drugs given to heart disease
patients.

Blood Builder (For anemia)

One of the most common malnutritive conditions in the world is iron deficiency anemia. Since iron is needed to make healthy red blood cells to deliver oxygen to all cells in the body, iron deficiency symptoms read like a patient who is slowly suffocating. These symptoms include fatigue, lethargy, confusion, irritability, gray skin (in extreme stages), and frequent infections.

- Take a drink made from 1 part red beet juice and 2 parts red grape juice. Take 1 T. 3–4 times daily. As a substitute, take beet powder capsules.

Other:

- The building of adequate red blood cells involves a host of nutrients including daily supplies—iron (10–30 mg), zinc (10–50 mg), copper (1–5 mg), B-12 (100–3000 mcg. may need to be intravenous or sublingual), folate (400–800 mcg), B-6 (5–50 mg), vitamin E to

prevent premature bursting of red blood cells (100–800 iu).[28]
Caution: excess iron stores have been shown to increase the risk for heart disease or cancer. Taking one mineral without a reasonable balance of other minerals can create a deficiency or imbalance.

Blood Clots

Following a typical modern lifestyle, blood has a tendency to become sticky and clump together, which creates numerous problems. Clots (thrombus) can get wedged in veins of the legs (phlebitis) or the brain (stroke). Sticky blood indicates a very serious problem, not just an inconvenient symptom. See your doctor.

• Take a few drops of juniper oil daily.

Other:

The stickiness of the blood is highly dependent on a set of body substances called prostaglandins. When we eat more sugar, saturated fat, hydrogenated fat, coupled with low intake of vitamin E; we are creating sticky blood cells that clot when they should not.

- Eat sweets in moderation and only with a mixed meal of protein, fat, and complex carbohydrates.
- Take 3–9 capsules/day of fish oil, or 1–3 T. of liquid fish oil to markedly reduce the stickiness of blood cells.[27]
- Take 2400 iu/day of mixed natural tocopherols of vitamin E from Grace Company (See Appendix).

There are numerous studies showing that taking
1–2 aspirin/day can reduce the stickiness of blood cells and hence the risk for cancer or heart disease. However, there are an equal number of studies showing that aspirin has many side effects, including intestinal bleeding which make it far from the "safe" drug it is called. I do not encourage the long term use of aspirin as a preventive agent.

Blood Purifier

The blood stream carries the "river of life" through 60,000 miles of vessels to feed all cells with nutrients and to carry away waste products to be excreted through lungs, kidneys, sweat pores, or colon. The blood, not unlike a river near a major city, is often full with toxic debris. When this toxic burden becomes excessive, a little herbal help may be in order.

- Take ¼ to ½ tsp. Epsom salts in a 6 oz. glass of lemonade before breakfast each morning. This will cleanse the blood, kidneys, and bowels.
- Drink 8 oz. of beet juice daily.
- Chew burdock seeds to cleanse the blood and eliminate boils and styes.
- Pour one c. of boiling water over 2 T. of the following herbal concoction: 4 parts dandelion root, 4 parts burdock, 4 parts red clover, 1 part fennel seed. Let steep, cool, strain. Drink 2 T. thirty minutes after meals.

- Cleansing fast. After a 1–3 day fast (consuming water only), drink ¼ c. unsweetened fruit or vegetable juice the first day and every 2 hours thereafter. Eating too much after a fast can be harmful and undo the benefits of the fast. You should be in good health. Diabetics should not attempt a fast.

- In place of breakfast, begin in the morning sipping from a 24-oz. container of unsweetened concord grape juice. Finish the juice by 10 a.m. Eat lunch and dinner as usual, excluding any form of pork. If your stomach cannot tolerate the grape juice, then dilute it and gradually build up the concentration. Continue this grape juice semi-fast program for 6 weeks.

Blood in Urine

- Drink tea from horsetail grass or comfrey root, but see a doctor first, since blood in the urine is worthy of concern.

Boils

- Lay the thin skin from the inside of a freshly broken eggshell on the sore.
- Twice daily, take 1 tsp. of blackstrap molasses sprinkled lightly with cream of tartar.
- Drink tea from burdock.
- Dip a hydrangea leaf in boiling water and apply to the boil.
- Apply finely chopped comfrey roots to the boil.
- Mix 4 oz. sublimed sulphur with 16 oz. honey. Take 1 tsp. internally at bedtime.
- Make a liniment from black ointment.
- Drink red clover blossom tea.
- Make a poultice from equal parts of linseed oil (special type), honey, and flour. Apply the poultice to the boil.
- Consume capsules of chaparral leaves. (See also section on Poultice for Green Mountain Salve).

Bruises

When you bump your flesh, you may break tiny blood vessels that spill blood into the surrounding tissue and leave the recognizable blue bruise. Some people bruise far too easily, which can be an indicator of overall poor health, in particular the inability to create tough collagen (connective tissue).

- Apply a cold wet rag immediately to the region to help prevent swelling and control pain.

Other:

Higher intakes of vitamin C has been shown to improve resistance to bruising.

- Recommendations: Take 2 grams/day of vitamin C the first day. Add 1 gram each day until reaching 12 grams/day. Use buffered vitamin C if regular vitamin C causes stomach upset.

Bioflavonoids, such as rutin and hesperidin, are accessory (helper) substances to facilitate the functions of vitamin C.

- Recommendation: Take 200–1000 mg of rutin daily with the vitamin C.

Another key missing ingredient in maintaining healthy connective tissue is zinc. Many Americans, particularly senior citizens, are low in zinc intake, which can lead to excessive bruising.

- Recommendation: Take 50–100 mg/day zinc picolinate.[29]

Burns

- For sunburn, bathe in cold water.

- Apply an ice pack.

- Apply the jelly from a freshly cut aloe plant.

- Dab the burn with a cooled tea made from cheese plant (common mallow).

- Apply honey directly to the burn, cut, or sore.

Bursitis

(See also Gout and Rheumatism.)

- Take 400–800 mg calcium supplements just as you feel the pain coming on.
- Apply vinegar to the sore area.
- Make a mixture of vinegar and water and drink to relieve bursitis.

Cancer

Basically, cancer is abnormal growth that has taken over the body's normal healthy processes. Cancer can grow like a parasite, strangling vital organs, draining the body of essential nutrients, and depressing the immune system until death usually comes from infection, organ failure, or malnutrition. Cancer is a life threatening disease which requires immediate medical attention. A successful approach to the treatment of cancer would include external medicine to reduce tumor burden, coupled with stimulation of the body's internal healing mechanisms. With your doctor's approval, you may want to consider some of the following therapies that augment your doctor's treatment.

- For centuries, the Amish have relied on 10–20 drops each morning of red clover to prevent cancer. Red clover is an ingredient in numerous other herbal remedies for cancer.
- For skin cancer, apply a poultice of the green flesh of the pipe organ cactus.

- For skin cancer, at night apply ⅓ grated fresh papaya bound in a sock and taped to the sore.

- For skin cancer, apply a poultice of crushed wood sorrel (oxalis) leaves.

- Drink a tea from Pau d'Arco bark that has been boiled for 10 minutes and then steeped for 10 more minutes.

- Eat 2 T. cooked asparagus daily.

- Drink a tonic made from 2 c. red clover blossoms, 1 c. berberis root (Rocky Mountain grape), ½ c. prickly ash root, 4 c. buckthorn, 2 c. alfalfa leaves, 1 c. pokeberry root, and ½ c. yellow dock root. Mix herbs and fill #00 gelatin capsules. Adults take 2 capsules after each meal and at bedtime (4 times daily).

- Drink 2–3 cups daily of Jason Winters' tea. (Mr. Winters developed brain cancer, then searched the world for herbal mixtures to help his otherwise untreatable condition. He now markets the herbal concoction that he feels led to his recovery.)

Chaparral plant:

- Drink chaparral tea mixed with crimson clover blossoms and aloe root.

- For skin cancer, apply a poultice of dried chaparral leaves.

- For skin cancers, melt ½ gallon hog's lard without salt in a large kettle. Drop a large handful of fresh green rue and let it grow brown. Beat up 9 eggs and add. When the mixture turns brown, discard the herbs and cool. Apply topically to suspicious areas.

- Boil 1 lb. fresh figs slowly in 1 gallon fresh cow's milk until figs are soft. Remove figs from mixture and stir in a separate container until figs develop poultice texture. Every 12 hours, apply a poultice of the figs and drink 1 c. of the remaining milk solution. Skin cancer should break open in 24–48 hours and then begin healing.

- Start by taking 1 drop of USP (United States Pharmacopoeia) iodine in a half glass of water after each meal. The second day, take 2 drops per dose. Each day add 1 extra drop until you have a warm or queer feeling in your stomach. Decrease the dose until you feel comfortable again. Continue this regimen.

- Create herbal concoction consisting of: 1 c. bloodroot, 2 c. red clover blossoms, 1 T. ginger. Add 1 quart of water and boil down to 1 pint. Strain and add 1 pint of whiskey. Take 1 tsp. 3 times/day.

- Many generations have used salves to treat skin cancer. One formula commercially available is Cansema, which includes a proprietary blend of zinc chloride, blood root, and chaparral. See sources in the Appendix for address.

Cataracts

- Scrape raw potato, put on cloth, and apply to the closed eyes. Leave on overnight. Or, press juice out of an old raw potato. With an eye dropper put two drops into each eye every evening before retiring. Make fresh juice each evening.
- Twice daily, bath eyes in warm salt water followed by warm vinegar water.

Other:

- Numerous clinicians are reporting reversal of cataracts with supplements that include high dose antioxidants: 800 iu vitamin E, 5 grams vitamin C, 15,000 iu beta-carotene, plus 30 mg zinc.[30]
- There is also good evidence that a diet low in calories, sugar, and dairy products coupled with optimal levels of various vitamins and minerals can prevent or delay the onset of cataracts.[31]

Circulation

- To improve circulation and warmth, soak feet in hot water with a bit of red pepper.
- Use inner soles in the shoes made of wool felt to keep feet warm.
- Drink a weak tea made from the leaves and flowers of the hawthorn berry (crataegus oxycantha).

Cayenne peppers:

- Eat cayenne peppers or fill small capsules with cayenne powder and take twice daily with plenty of fluid.
- Boil a one inch section of bloodroot in 1 c. of water for a few minutes. Take 1 T. each day.
- Drink tansy tea 3–4 times daily.

Colds

- Take vitamins A & D throughout the winter to prevent colds.
- To warm the throat and make a hostile environment for the germs, gargle with hot salt water, spit it out. Repeat in 15 minutes.
- To both prevent and help cure colds, cut open a fresh onion and lay it out on the kitchen shelf.
- Boil a pot of water with peppermint oil or pine oil so the house occupants will inhale the vapors.
- Rub the outside of the throat glands with camphor or Vicks, then cover with flannel cloth.
- Drink lots of herbal teas, unsweetened juices, lemon tea, or hot chicken broth.
- Place a drop of peppermint oil in a bowl of boiling water with the face held close to inhale the vapors.
- Place a drop of peppermint oil in a tsp. of brown sugar and swallow.

- Place a drop of peppermint oil on a handkerchief and place to the nose before retiring in the evening.

- For children, place a drop of peppermint oil on their pillowcase at night before sleeping.

- Drink sage tea.

- Give children (over 2 years) a tsp. of honey before putting them to bed to help them breath easier.

- Place a drop of salt water solution (8 oz. water with ½ tsp. salt) in the nostrils, or use nasal purge as described in "allergy" section.

- Take 1 T. daily of cod liver oil to build resistance.

- To break a fever, juice ½ lemon, fill a glass with water, add ½ tsp. of bicarbonate of soda. Drink this solution every half hour until fever breaks.

- Drink hot lemon tea with honey. Juice ½ lemon for each cup of tea.

- When first symptoms of flu appear, take 1 tsp. of vinegar, a sprinkle of bicarbonate of soda, red pepper, and ginger in ½ c. of warm water.

- Boil 1 gallon of dandelion flowers in 1 gallon of water for 5 minutes. Let stand for 3 days in a glass jug or stainless steel container. Strain, then boil the peelings of 2 lemons and 1 orange in the dandelion water for 15 minutes. Let stand until lukewarm. Slice in the 2 lemons and 1 orange. Add 2 tsp. yeast and 3 lb. sugar. Cover with cloth and let stand 6 days. Bottle. When having a cold, take 1 T. at bedtime or as needed.

Other:

High doses of vitamin C have been shown to lower the incidence, duration, and severity of colds.[32]

- Recommendation: take 1–5 grams of vitamin C daily, and 1 gram/hour if you have a cold.

Zinc lozenges have been shown to reduce the duration and intensity of a cold.[33]

- Recommendations: Take 1 zinc lozenge (15 mg. zinc) every 3 hours while having a cold.

Cold Sores

Herpes simplex is a nasty virus that seems to permanently reside in certain unfortunate individuals. It is spread by mucus in people who are genetically vulnerable. It flares up in times of emotional or physical stress.

- Drink sage tea.

Other:

- Vitamin C supplements (1–2 grams) virtually eliminated flare-ups in 30 of 38 cold sore patients.[34]
- Bioflavonoid supplements (1000–1500 mg) helped 2/3 of herpes subjects.[35]
- Topical vitamin E provided pain relief for herpes sores.[36]
- L-lysine (1–6 grams) tripled the recovery rate for

    herpes patients.[37]

Colic

- Make a tea by boiling 1 c. water with 1 tsp. fennel seeds. Cool to lukewarm, strain.
- Prepare a tea from chamomile and/or catnip.
- Give peppermint or spearmint tea.
- To remove sour vomit odor, fill a container with baking soda and place in room.

Other:

- If the nursing mother discontinues eating dairy products (milk, cheese, ice cream, etc.), then she may see a dramatic improvement in her child's colic. The child's allergy to cow's milk is caused by mother's consumption of milk products.
- Change formula from cow's milk to goat milk, which is closer in nutrient content to human milk.

Colon Problems

(constipation, colitis)

- Eat more roughage, which includes unprocessed fruits, vegetables, whole grains, and beans. A favorite Amish cereal recipe: 6 cups oatmeal, 1 c. shredded coconut, 3 c. wheat germ, ½ c. chopped almonds, ½ c. chopped pecans, 1.5 c. brown sugar, ½ tsp. salt, ½ c. vegetable oil. Mix in big bowl then toast until crunchy.
- Teas made from senna leaf, or flaxseed, or psyllium seed help.
- Chew well then swallow 1 tsp. flaxseed.
- Take magnesium supplements (400 mg. daily) or take 1 tsp. Epsom salts with glass of warm water.
- Get more exercise, which helps the muscles of the abdomen move the food to the colon.
- May be caused by too many gravies, pastries, breads, and not enough exercise.
- Avoid white flour and fried foods.

- Drink at least 6 glasses daily of purified water. Sprinkle in some powdered vitamin C to neutralize cancer-causing nitrates in the stomach.
- Sprinkle 1 tsp. ground flaxseed on your cereal each morning. Or boil the flax seeds then strain and drink the tea.
- For lower bowel problems, use enema of either 8 oz. lukewarm black coffee, or warm salt water solution (8 oz. water with ½ tsp. sea salt).
- Boil flax seeds in water, strain, then drink the tea.
- Drink a glass of hot water on rising in the morning.
- Skip a meal or two, then drink unsweetened juices for a half a day or longer.
- Give your organs a rest by eating less. Eat plenty of raw salads and fruits.
- Take 1 tsp. ground psyllium seeds in ½ c. unsweetened juice in the morning upon arising and in the evening. In the morning

follow with a large capsule filled with Epsom salts. Continue for 2 weeks.

- To make your own suppositories, mix 1 oz. each of goldenseal, boric acid, white flour in with glycerine until stiff. Form into suppositories and refrigerate. When needed, insert in rectum at bedtime and leave until morning.

- Consume only unlimited amounts of grape juice for 3 days.

- Take 1 tsp. powdered psyllium seed with fruit juice about 15 minutes before breakfast.

- Put one rounded tsp. of slippery elm powder into a glass with hot milk. This may be used on cereal. Follow this procedure in the evening and every day until relieved. Psyllium seed cleanses the colon and slippery elm aids healing.

- Drink 1–2 c. golden seal tea. Take a gulp every few hours during the day for 2 weeks. Quit a few days occasionally, then continue.

- Drink a quart of peppermint tea daily, sweetened with honey.

- Use enemas with warm water tea made from burdock roots or inner white oak bark. Use 2 T. of root or bark to 1.5 quarts of water. Let brew, then cool to desired temperature. Strain through cloth. Take one high enema daily for 6 days, then only occasionally as needed.

- Make a drink from 1/4 tsp. powdered myrrh and 1/4 tsp. golden seal in ½ glass of very warm water. Also take 5 grams of garlic capsules 3 times/day.

- Avoid cold water, sugar, pastries, onions, black pepper, and pickled foods.

- Olive oil, prune juice, buttermilk, or yogurt in the diet will prevent and treat constipation.

- To relieve diarrhea of colitis: boil wild blackberry root or red oak bark in water and drink ½ c. If not relieved drink another ½ c. in several hours.

- Take 1 T. of safflower oil each day to heal the lining of the colon.

- Take 1 T. of flaxseed oil (dietary linseed oil) to speed healing of the colon.

- For piles, drink a tea from sumac tops before bedtime and upon arising; or apply a poultice of jimson weeds fried in lard and spread on area.
- For relief from piles, steam the affected part by sitting over a pan containing garlic boiled in milk.

Other:

- Many diseases are precipitated by constipation. Regularity is a hallmark of a healthy body. Typically, a diet high in fiber (food from plants) and water will provide excellent regularity for most individuals. Some people may need to add supplements of fiber to encourage daily bowel movements. Laxatives and enemas should be used sparingly, as they can be habit forming and make the bowels lazy.
- Assist the muscles of the intestines by stomach massaging. Do this by using the palm side of a closed fist to rock gently over the intestinal area. This helps to move the

fecal matter through the intestines for elimination.

- An excellent laxative is high doses of vitamin C. Many experts feel that the ideal intake of vitamin C is just below "bowel tolerance", or the level which causes diarrhea. For most healthy adults, this "bowel tolerance" is in the range of 10–20 grams/day. The high doses of C provide many benefits in the system, while helping to encourage regularity in the bowels.[38]

Corns

- Soak a small piece of cloth in vinegar. Bind it on the toe, leaving it on day and night. The corn will come out by the root.
- For corns, soak feet in warm water for 15 minutes, then apply the inside of a small piece of lemon peel to the corn and tape it there overnight. After three nights, the corn should lift out.

Cough

- Mix equal parts of lemon juice, honey, and castor oil. Adults take 1 T/day and children over 2 years old take 1 tsp./day.
- Steep ½ tsp. dried crushed green peach tree leaves in 1 quart boiling water for 10 minutes. Take 1 T. of this tea every hour with a few drops of honey.
- Steep 4 chestnut leaves in 1 pint boiling water. Sweeten with honey and drink 5–6 times daily.
- Boil one lemon, squeeze out the juice, add 1 c. honey. Take 1–2 T. at bedtime or as needed.
- Drink fenugreek tea to eliminate mucus.
- Make a cough syrup by washing mullein leaves, boil for 10 minutes, add enough sugar for flavor, then boil down to a thick syrup.
- Use vinegar as a gargle to help clear up a cough.
- Gargle with hot salt water or hot sumac tea.

- Drink a tea made from slippery elm bark and horehound.
- Peel and slice onions. Fry them until brown. Place these tolerably warm onions between two large clean washcloths or handkerchiefs and lay on the chest for a poultice.
- Apply Po Ho oil to chest.
- To make cough drops, mix 1 oz. cubeb powder, 2 oz. gum arabic, 2 oz. licorice root powdered, and 1 lb. powdered sugar with 4 T. water.
- To make a cough syrup, mix 8 oz. of honey with 7 drops of eucalyptus oil (or cherry bark) and stir well. Take a few drops when needed.
- To make a cough syrup, cut 1 lb. of fresh garlic into slices. Add garlic to 1 quart boiling water in jar, cover, and let stand for 12 hours. Boil 1 tsp. each of: bruised caraway and fennel seeds in 4 oz. vinegar; then strain and add to garlic mixture. Add honey for flavor and give 1–2 T. when needed.
- Rub the chest, back, and throat with goose fat.

- A swallow of pineapple juice on regular basis helps.

- Mix 2 T. brown sugar, 1 T. butter, 2 T. vinegar. Heat until melted. Blend. While still warm, serve 1 tsp. to patient.

- Inhale the warm vapors from a bath or shower of hot water. Loosens the mucus in the throat and lungs.

- Steep 1/3 c. horehound with 1 tsp. sassafras in 1 quart boiling water for 10–15 minutes. Strain, then add 1/4 c. honey. Take a swallow or two when bothered.

- Put 1 oz. lobelia in a pint of boiling water. Cool. Take 2 T. every 4 hours.

- Mix 1/4 oz. lobelia, black cohosh root, and chestnut leaves in a jar. Pour ½ pint boiling water on the herbs and let stand for 30 minutes. Strain, then add 1 lb. sugar and bring to a boil. Remove scum and give 1 tsp. every hour to children.

- Simmer one thinly sliced lemon and ½ pint flaxseed in 1 quart water for 4 hours. Strain while hot. Add 2 oz. honey. Take 1 T. three times daily or more after severe coughing session.

Cramps

- For a "charley horse", drink at least a quart of milk/day.
- Eat 4–8 soda crackers/day.
- Drink 1 tsp. of vinegar/day.
- Rub olive oil on the sole of the foot.
- Soak the feet in hot water.
- For general cramps, drink a hot tea made with 1/4 tsp. ginger.
- Drink a hot tea made with thyme.
- For monthly female cramps, make a poultice from catnip and rub on the abdomen.

Deodorant

- Mix 1 T. vegetable oil, 2 T. cornstarch, 2 T. bicarbonate of soda in a small pan heated on stove until blended. Store in small container and apply as deodorant.

Other:

- The body's odor is reflective of what is happening inside. Strong foul odors from the skin indicates illness, poor diet, or toxin buildup.
- Easiest way to eliminate body odor is to eliminate the place that most bacteria can buildup: shave the hairs in the armpit. You will not need deodorant.
- Realize that many deodorants either block pores to reduce the outlets for poisons, or worse yet some contain aluminum which can be absorbed by the skin and buildup into Alzheimer's disease.
- Eat less fat and less red meat for a sweeter smell.

- Sweat at least once each day, preferably by exercise, but also by hot showers and tubs to keep the skin pores flushed out. There are 3500 sweat pores per postage-stamp-sized space on your skin. Altogether, you have 40 miles of pores that need to be flushed and drained often.

Diabetes

In addition to following your doctor's directions, you may want to consider the following:

- Drink 3 cups daily of tea from boiling 1/4 avocado leaf, 1 eucalyptus leaf, and 1 walnut leaf.
- Drink a tea from peach leaf (1 leaf per c.).
- Drink a tea from marshmallow (cheese plant).
- Take capsules containing the following combination: cedar berries, uva ursi, licorice root, mullein, cayenne, and golden seal root.
- Drink tea from strawberry leaf or Pau d'Arco to lower blood sugar levels.

- Drink tea from arrowbruce or blueberry leaf to stimulate pancreatic health.
- Eat artichokes like apples.
- Kelp (seaweed, or sea vegetables) in the diet often helps.
- Plenty of oatmeal and dried beans help the diabetic.
- Drink tea made from clover blossoms and dandelions.
- Drink tea made from cheese plant (kas bobbla).

Other:

- There is plenty of scientific evidence showing that most diabetics can be helped through nutrition, while some can be "cured". Reduce body fat. Eat less refined carbohydrates, including white sugar and white flour. Take daily supplements of chromium picolinate (400–600 mcg), carnitine (1–2 grams), B-6 (50–100 mg), vitamin E (2,000 iu), zinc (30–50 mg), inositol ("muscle sugar" 1–2 grams), ginseng (500 mg), and eat fenugreek (a leguminous plant) often.[39]

Diaper Rash

- Apply vitamin E ointment to trouble area.
- Rub Vaseline® over the entire diaper area before putting the baby to bed in the evening.
- For prickly heat, rub the affected parts with the inside of watermelon rind. Or sponge with equal parts of water and vinegar.
- Apply ointment containing vitamins A & D.
- Be sure to dry diapers in sunlight after washing them to eliminate fungus.
- Apply cornstarch when changing diapers.

Diarrhea

- Drink tea made from caraway seeds.
- Eat ½ c. blueberries.

- Brew tea from either: slippery elm, or blackberry, or dried blackberry roots, or red raspberry leaf, or white oak bark.

- Drink tea made from leaves of green soup-bean plant.

- Bring 1 c. of milk to a boil. Add 1 tsp. nutmeg, 1/8 tsp. cinnamon, and honey. Drink at mealtime instead of eating heavy food.

- Mix 1 tsp. flour with 1 tsp. nutmeg, 1 tsp. white sugar, and pinch of salt in glass. Add enough water to make easy to drink. Take every 4 hours.

- For children, give 2 tsp. vinegar every 2 hours.

- Boil carrots, then puree. Take 1 tsp. every 15 minutes.

- Cook rice until soft. For infants, give rice water with a bit of sugar and milk. For older children, eat the whole rice.

- Mix ½ c. fresh orange juice, 1 T. sugar, 1/6 tsp. salt, 1 1/3 c water. Give child ½ oz. of this every 2 hours.

- Summertime diarrhea may be brought on by drinking too much cold fluids.
- Drink boneset tea.
- Mix ½ oz. each of skullcap, feverfew, and lady slipper. Place in quart jar, then fill with boiling water, let steep for 2 hours. Take 2 T. three times daily.
- Drink tea from black snake grass roots.

Digestion and Stomach Problems

- To purge the body of amoebic parasites, make a tea from 1 tsp. mango tree bark in 1 c. boiling water.

- To purge the body of parasites, eat 1 papaya leaf daily or take 3–6 garlic capsules daily.

- To rid the body of worms, mix this anti-parasitic syrup: fennel seed, black walnut hulls, senna leaves, male fern, tansey, tame sage, and wormwood.

- Drink a tea from pumpkin seeds to rid the body of parasites.

Dropsy

- Boil 6 one inch pieces of Christ root in 2 c. water for 5 minutes. Take 1 T. several times daily.
- Drink a tea of horsetail grass, stinging nettle, rosemary, and birch leaves.
- Mix 1 gallon pure apple cider, 1 handful of horseradish, 2 handfuls of parsley, 2 T. mustard seeds, 1 oz. juniper berries. Let stand in a warm place for 24 hours, strain, then drink 2 T. 4–5 times daily.

Earache

(in children, or if persists, then see a doctor)

- Use fresh sheep wool with lanolin still intact. Make a wad and put in ears.
- Place a cold wet wash rag on ears.
- To relieve pain, dip cotton wad in molasses and stuff into ears.
- Add a few drops of Oil of Herbs to the ears.

- Use otagesine, product available in health food stores.
- Mix 1 T. each olive oil with oil of rue and place several drops in the ears.
- Rub olive oil, or herb oil, or Vicks on the area surrounding the ears.
- Gather small mullein (wool draut) flowers. Put them in a bottle and place in the sun. The flowers emit an oil. Put 1–2 drops of the oil in the ears then plug with cotton.

Eczema

- Apply a paste made from lard and sulphur to the affected region. Make sure to wear old clothes over the sulphur-lard, since this ruins clothes.
- Eat 2 T. brewer's yeast daily.
- Apply vitamin E liquid to the affected skin.
- Apply a salve of emulsified fish oil to the skin. Cover with flannel and tape on.
- Drink goat's milk.

Endurance, Energy

(see also "tonic")

- Mix 1 T. each of finely chopped yellow dock, burdock, dandelion, black snake root, and sassafras bark into a jar of wine and let stand for 3 months. Take one T. each morning before breakfast.
- Drink tansy tea often.
- Soak 1 T. chia seeds overnight in a c. of water, strain, and drink liquid in the morning.
- An afternoon nap of 30 minutes is equal in sleep value to 2 hours at night.

Eyes

- Drink tea made from eyebright or goldenseal herbs.
- To improve eye health, take 6–10 capsules daily of carrot seed oil.
- Growth of cataracts can be retarded by adding 1 drop of flaxseed oil in eyes at bedtime.

- Use elderberry blossom tea as an eye wash to cure pink eye.
- Warm chamomile tea dropped into eyes will cure styes.
- If you have a tiny irritant in the eye, then put a single flaxseed under the eyelid. The irritant will be drawn to the seed, which should be removed shortly.

Female Problems

(Menopause: change of life)

- Drinking a tea made from chestnut leaves was known to be good for this trouble.
- Create a herbal tea concoction from rosemary, horsetail, grass, yarrow, shepherd's purse, dwarf elder, peppermint. Drink 2 cups/day, with a swallow now and again.

Other:

- A female gynecologist has found tremendous success with her clients by giving

2,000 iu/day vitamin E to relieve hot flashes.[40]

Fertility

- For both men and women, consume 1 T. daily of both carrot seed oil and wheat germ oil.
- Eat a diet rich in alfalfa sprouts.
- Abstain from working around pesticides and other questionable chemicals.
- Men should avoid wearing tights pants and heavy cotton underwear as this added warmth cuts down on sperm count.
- Pumpkin seeds or 50 mg/day of zinc supplements can help men.

Other:

- Excellent studies show that fertility in women can be improved by: maintaining proper weight, avoiding caffeine and alcohol, taking supplements of B-6 (100–300 mg). Fertility for men can be improved by: avoiding alcohol, taking B-12 (6000 mcg), vitamin C (1–2 grams), zinc (30–60 mg), and L-arginine (4 grams).[41]

Fever

- Make a paste with flour and vinegar. Spread on a cloth and apply to the bottom of the patient's feet.
- Beat one egg white with 1 tsp. sugar and 1/4 c. water. Drink this solution.
- Make tea from the bark of weeping willow tree. Simmer for 5 minutes. Add willow leaves, then steep for at least 15 minutes. Take 1 tsp. of this tea washed down with 1 c. water. Dilute for children.
- Drink tea from pennyroyal, lobelia, or red clover (½ tsp. per c. water).
- Drink tea from strawberry leaf, or alfalfa, or yarrow.

Fish Bone Stuck in Throat

(After calling "911" emergency number)

- Gargle with vinegar or take a few swallows of strong vinegar, which may soften the bones.
- Break an egg into a glass and have them swallow it.

Other:

- Try to dislodge obstruction by thumping on back or turning upside down, or grabbing around waist just below the rib cage and forcefully squeezing.

Flu

- To relieve chest congestion, mix a salve of 6 oz. sheep tallow, 15 oz. valeine, 3 oz. menthol crystals, 3 oz. beeswax; then melt and add 2 oz. gum camphor oil, 2 oz. sassafras oil, 2 oz. eucalyptus oil. Apply this mixture liberally to the chest.

- Special remedy for children: make a large pot of tea from Queen Anne's lace and use this for a hot foot bath for children while draping their body with warm wool blankets. At the same time, have the children drink elder blossom tea.

- Drink a tea from elderberry flowers.

- Drink a tea from 1/4 tsp. cayenne in 1 c. hot water. Encourages the body to sweat.

- Drink a tea from equal parts bayberry bark, ginger root, cloves, cayenne, and white pine bark.

- Drink a tea from 1 lb. bayberry bark, 1 lb. ginger root, 2 oz. cayenne pepper, 2 oz. cloves. Finely pulverize and mix ingredients. Mix 1/4 tsp. of herbal concoction with 1 tsp. sugar in a cup of boiling water. Let stand and drink.

Frostbite

- Mix 1 oz. each of olive oil, peppermint oil, and ammonia and rub on frostbitten hands.
- Soak frostbitten hands in cold water. Rub hands but do not hold directly to heat.

Gallbladder and Gallstones

- Take 1 tsp. parsley juice every morning upon arising.
- Take the juice of 1–2 lemons before retiring at night. Drink undiluted, then lie on right side for 20 minutes.
- Juice 3 lemons, add 3 tsp. cream of tartar, 3 tsp. Epsom salts. Put in pint jar of water. Take 1 T. of this solution each morning before breakfast.

- Take 1 tsp. olive oil followed immediately by 1 tsp. lemon juice. Do this three times daily for 3 consecutive days while fasting.
- Drink a solution of 6 oz. olive oil with 6 oz. pure lemon juice to eliminate gallstones.

- For gallstones, drink a gallon of pure apple juice for two consecutive days, averaging 1 c./hour. Fast for these 2 days. On the third morning, begin with drinking 4 oz. pure cold pressed olive oil. Gradually return to solid foods. May also help kidney stones.
- Eat only grapefruit or grapefruit juice until relieved.
- Before retiring, take 6 oz olive oil with a bit of water. First thing in the morning, take 1 tsp. Epsom salts with some water.
- Make a tea from 10 tsp. ground root of sweet weed and ½ tsp. sacred bark boiled in 1 pint of water for 1 hour. Strain through cheesecloth and cool. Consume ½ c. daily until relief comes.

Gas (Flatulence)

- Swallow 2 capsules daily of ginger root, or drink hot ginger tea, or homemade ginger ale.

- Chew 1 tsp. of coriander seeds or caraway seeds.
- Drink warm mint tea with meals.
- Eat slowly. Food consumed quickly has many trapped pockets of gas.
- Avoid carbonated drinks, like soda pop.
- Mix the following herbs and take capsules at dinner time: fennel, wild yam, catnip, ginger, peppermint, spearmint, papaya, and lobelia.

Gout

- Apply a poultice of chopped fresh onions daily.
- Eat a diet with 2 cups fresh cherries and no meat.
- Take capsules with yucca and devil's claw leaves.

Hair and Skin Care

Hair:

- Use Vel® bar soap (or castile soap) to shampoo hair and vinegar to rinse the hair.
- Beat egg whites and apply to the scalp. Let stand for 3 minutes. Rinse well.
- Add several drops of baby oil (mineral oil) to the hair rinse solution for better managed hair.
- Shampoo with a mixture of rosemary leaves, chamomile leaves, rosewater, and mild soap. Can add 1 beaten egg with natural coconut oil to this mixture.

Baldness:

- For baldness, consume 40 drops daily of red clover tops liquid extract. Use a scalp rinse of vinegar with sage tea.
- Take 30–60 mg supplemental zinc daily.

- Rub aloe vera into the scalp for thinning hair.

Dandruff:

- Rub a small amount of pure coconut oil in the scalp daily.
- Use tea from burdock or sage as a scalp rinse after shampoo.
- Dissolve 1 tsp. borax (boric acid) in 1 c. water. Using a brush, wet the hair with this solution every day for a week, then twice each week for 3 weeks.
- Mix ½ oz sulphur in a pint of water. Let stand for 2 days while shaking occasionally. Dampen the scalp 3–4 times/week with this solution.
- Gather stinging nettles with gloves on. Boil 1 c stinging nettles in 1 pint of water and add 1 T vinegar. Cool and strain. Use this tea for rinsing the hair.

Skin:

- Mix 1/4 c. olive oil with 1 tsp. sugar and massage hands twice weekly with solution.
- Mix 1 oz glycerine, 1 oz rubbing alcohol, 1 oz camphor spirit, 1 oz of 10% ammonia and use this solution for a hand creme.
- For a lotion to heal dry skin, mix 4 oz. glycerine, 4 oz. alcohol, 1 oz. quince seed. First pour one pint boiling water on quince seed and let soak overnight, then strain and add other ingredients.
- Apply a mixture of equal parts bay rum and glycerine.
- Make a paste of cornstarch and evaporated milk. Apply to face and throat. Let dry. Bath with cold water to remove.
- For dry skin, mix together a salve of equal parts of cocoa butter, glycerine, lanolin, rosewater, and elderflower water.
- For eczema, gather black poplar buds (balm of Gilead) in the spring when buds are sticky, boil in olive oil, strain, make a salve.

- Make herbal capsules from equal parts barberry, wild yam, cramp bark, fennel seed, ginger, catnip, and peppermint. Take 2 capsules 15 minutes before bedtime.
- For white spots on skin, make a salve of hog lard, limes, and sulphur.

Scar Tissue:

- To help prevent scar tissue from forming, repeatedly rub cocoa butter on wound.
- To help prevent scarring, apply vitamin E ointment to wound.
- To help dissolve scar tissue, rub on castor oil

Freckling:

- To reduce freckling, bathe the face in fresh buttermilk. Or mix 2 oz. sour milk with 2 drams grated horseradish, 6 drams cornmeal; spread this mixture between thin muslin and apply to affected parts at night, making sure not to get into eyes.

Headache

Often caused by stress. Learn the art of relaxation.

- Take 1/4 tsp. soda in a c. of warm water before going to bed and upon arising.
- Using forefinger pressure, massage the back of the neck.
- Saturate a cloth in ice cold vinegar, squeeze out excess, then bind around forehead.
- Soak feet for 10–20 minutes in a hot foot bath of water and 2 tsp. powdered mustard. At the same time, apply a handkerchief well dampened with equal parts of water and vinegar to the forehead.

- Apply oil of rosemary lotion at the temples. Gently massage into skin, keeping away from the eyes.

Other:

- The herb feverfew has been demonstrated effective in the treatment of migraine headaches.[42]

Heart and Blood Pressure

- For irregular heart beat mix 1 tsp. each of black cohosh, skullcap, valerian, lobelia, and cayenne in 1 pint of boiling water. Drink 1–2 cups of this tea daily.
- The Amish eat an apple a day to keep the doctor away, and plenty of garlic each day to keep everybody else away!
- Vitamin E, C, and lecithin are advised for the heart. Many Amish men take 100–300 iu daily of vitamin E. Whole wheat bread can add substantially to vitamin E intake.

- Avoid excess of high cholesterol foods, including eggs, bacon, ham, butter, cheese, ice cream, milk (except for children), and chocolate.
- Daily consume a tea made from Hawthorn berries and cayenne (red pepper).
- Teas made from sassafras, burdock, or red clover help to thin and cleanse the blood.
- Exercise helps to prevent heart attacks. Walk daily. A mini-trampoline in the home can be helpful.
- Teas from rosemary, chamomile, or red pepper before retiring each night help to improve circulation.

- Phlebitis (inflammation of the veins) can be relieved by taking 1 tsp. safflower oil before breakfast, 3 garlic oil capsules before meals, 3 cups alfalfa seed tea daily (2 tsp. crushed seeds in 1 c. boiling water). Also, to relieve the pain of phlebitis, apply a salve of ginseng, aloe vera, allantoin, vitamins A, D, E, and B-6.

- Palpitations of the heart can be caused by gas upset in the stomach, which can be relieved by drinking 8 oz water with ½ tsp. bicarbonate of soda.

- Ten minutes before breakfast, mix 1 T. honey with 3 tsp. vinegar in 8 oz. warm water and drink.

- For high blood pressure, mix ½ tsp. cream of tartar, 2 T. sulphur, and 2 T. Epsom salts in 1 quart water. Shake well and take 2 T. daily.
- Garlic, lecithin, and asparagus help control blood pressure.
- Mix 2 tsp. cider vinegar with 1 tsp. honey in 8 oz water and drink 10 minutes before bedtime.
- Avoid lard, fatty foods, margarine, shortening, and peanuts. Or eat nothing but unsweetened fruit for 2 days.
- Sesame seeds help to prevent fatty buildup in the arteries. Make a useful candy by mixing sesame seeds with a small amount of honey, form into balls, and keep in freezer.

Other:

In a 17 year study of thousands of people, researchers found that the most important nutritional predictor of heart disease was the
amount of vitamin E in the blood. Vitamin E
helps to prevent the "rusting" of fats, which
eventually block the arteries and lead to heart
disease. A diet high in fiber, green and orange
vegetables, and whole grains will lower the
risk for heart disease. Daily supplements of: vitamin E (300–800 iu), vitamin C (1–5 grams),
garlic (6 capsules), fish oil (1 T. oil), and chromium picolinate (400 mcg) will dramatically
lower the risk for, and, in some cases, even reverse heart disease.[43]

Hemorrhoids and Piles

- To a hot sitz bath, add 1 lb. alum.
- Apply a poultice from marigold, malva, comfrey, red clover, burdock, elder, and yellow
  dock.

- May be caused by eating too much grape-fruit.
- Omit pork from the diet for relief.
- Eat raw red beets between meals.

Other:

- Use toilet paper soaked in warm water to cleanse yourself, then dry toilet paper to dry yourself. This method alone virtually eliminates hemorrhoid pain in most people. Keep a cup of water by the toilet, or bring a warmed cup of water with you into the bathroom.

Hiccups

- Take a few rapid swallows of canned pine-apple juice. Repeat each hour if necessary.
- Just drinking water may help.
- Add 1/3 tsp. cream of tartar to 8 oz. warm water. Drink 2 T. at a time on empty stomach.
- Eat 1 tsp. peanut butter.
- Drink the juice from ½ orange.
- Hold the breath as long as you can.
- Take a tsp. of honey.

Other:

- Place a paper bag over your head, crimping the bag around the neck with your hands but allowing circulation in the throat region. Breath 4–5 times in a relaxed even method, then remove bag. Using the bag helps to equalize the ratio between carbon dioxide (exhaled) and oxygen (inhaled) in the bloodstream.

Hives

- Each morning drink a blend of ½ tsp. soda, ½ tsp. tartar, and 1 tsp. Epsom salts in 4 oz water.
- Steep catnip leaves in boiling water for 10 minutes. Strain, then wash the hives with the solution.

Ingrown Toenail

- Do not trim too far down on the sides of the toenail.
- Put peroxide on sore spot to cleanse.
- Soak the feet at least once daily in hot water.
- Cut a V-shape out of the front center of the toenail to find relief from toenail pain.

Insect Bites and Bee Stings

- Make a poultice paste of equal parts bicarbonate of soda and vinegar.
- Apply a fresh cut onion to the sting.
- Make a poultice by mixing 2 oz. olive oil, 1 dram carbolic acid, 1 dram pennyroyal, 1 dram cedar oil, 2 drams citronella oil, 2 drams tincture of camphor, and ½ dram acetic acid. Apply to bites to lessen sting, or as an insect repellent.

- To relieve itching, rub a moistened bar of soap on the sting.
- As an insect repellent, apply citronella on skin. Helps pets, too.
- Remove the stinger by laying a paring knife flat against the skin. Slide the sharp edge against the skin to draw it out. Do not try to pick it out with fingers as this will only spread the poison. Once stinger is out, bruise a plantain and rub into the sting.
- Dissolve 1/4 tsp. meat tenderizer in 1 tsp. water and rub into the skin around the sting.
- To keep insects away, keep an infusion of chamomile flowers in a bottle throughout the summertime and apply to the skin before going outdoors.
- To ease pain, rub one raw potato, lemon slice, poppy leaves, marigold, a slice of raw onion, or nasturtium leaves on the sting.
- Apply a poultice of ground saffron tea to the sting.

- Apply a poultice of baking soda and water to the sting.

Other:

- Make a poultice from chewing tobacco or shredded cigars with warm water. Form a thick paste. Apply to the insect sting. Has been known to even reverse allergic reactions to stings.

Electrical energy tends to neutralize or "denature" the poisonous proteins from stings and bites. For particularly dangerous snake and spider bites, use an electric "stun gun" to the injured area with electrodes on either side of the bite. Not for small children, but has been known to neutralize potentially lethal bites.

Insomnia

- Cultivate beautiful thoughts, especially in the evening. Listen to music or read poetry.

- Soak 1 tsp. plain gelatin in 1 c. boiling water. Then stir until mixed. Take 2 tsp. at supper time.
- Near bedtime, soak feet in hot water with 1/4 c. vinegar added.
- The following herbs in capsule or tea form may help: hops, vervain, valerian, skullcap, catnip, peppermint, and golden seal.
- Take 1–2 tsp. honey before retiring.
- Drink a glass of warm milk before bedtime.
- Many a mother has given catnip tea to babies to help them rest.

Other:

- In scientific studies on humans, valerian has been shown to improve sleep patterns without inducing any "hangover" effect.[44]

Itching

- Cover the itch with a poultice of cornstarch and let it dry on the skin.

- Apply witch hazel or rubbing alcohol.
- Add 1 tsp. soda to 1 quart of water and wash itch area.
- Place 3 cups cooked oatmeal in a cheese-cloth bag and soak in warm water for 15 minutes. Then use bag to rub over itch.

Kidney and Bladder

- Drink teas made from one or more of the following: nettle, yarrow (schaf ribbe), broom grass (gravel grass), burdock (gletta), dandelion root, and golden seal. Dried and roasted dandelion root can be used as a coffee substitute.
- To reduce fluid retention, drink tea made from corn silk.
- To help pass kidney stones, drink cucumber juice.
- To help in kidney stones, drink tea from ½ avocado leaf.

- For kidney problems, steep 3 tsp. brown corn seed in a pint of water and drink 1 c. daily.
- To help painlessly pass a kidney stone, eat no food but consume large amounts of unsweetened apple juice.
- Make a tea from 3 avocado leaves in one c. boiling water, steeped for 10 minutes.
- Vinegar tea or cranberry juice may help some people.
- Boil 1 tsp. of flaxseed in 1 c. water. Steep until lukewarm, then drink a cupful every 3–4 hours.
- Brew 3 T. peeled or cut up pumpkin seeds in 1 quart water for several hours. Drink ½ c. twice a day until relief is found.

Other:

- Bladder infections (cystitis) are more likely in women and can be difficult to treat with continuous antibiotics. Cranberries, cranberry juice, and now a pill with extract of

cranberry (See Appendix) can be used to
safely eliminate urinary tract infections.[45]

Leg Ulcers

- Apply a poultice of powdered sugar, lanolin, and tincture of benzoin. Massage the leg to improve circulation, rubbing upward.

Liver

- Cook 5 medium size red beets in a quart of water. Drink the beet water and eat the beets (unpickled). Or boil the juice down to a smaller quantity and take a T. each morning before breakfast.

Low Blood Pressure

- Fill a quart jar with finely diced beets, then add wine or whisky to the top of jar. Let stand 24 hours in warm place. Take 1–2 T. of this fluid twice daily.
- Eat plenty of fresh greens and red beets.
- Use blackstrap molasses often.

Lung

- Take 1–2 capsules cayenne pepper with food in stomach to relieve pain of pleurisy.
- For pneumonia, make a chest salve by melting ½ lb. Vaseline®, 2 oz. gum camphor, ½ tsp. carbolic acid, and 1 T. beeswax. Another formula for chest salve: melt 6 oz. lard, 2 oz. pulverized camphor, and 3 oz. beeswax; followed by 3 oz. white resin, 2 oz. red balsam of Peru, 2 drams oil of cedar while stirring often. Apply this salve until begins to itch, then wash off with rubbing alcohol.
- Apply a poultice of equal parts flaxseed meal with ground black mustard to the chest.
- Drink hot pennyroyal tea.

Measles

- Eyes get weak during measles. Rest in a dark room and do not read.
- Boil a cup of oats in 4 cups of water for 15 minutes. Strain and sweeten. Drink at cool temperature.
- Drink tea made from yarrow.

Memory

- Eat hazel nuts for 9 days. On the first day eat 6 nuts. Then add one additional nut each day.
- Eat green pepper seeds for 9 days. Begin with 1 seed the first day and double the dose until it reaches 256 seeds on the ninth day.
- Make a paste of ground cloves, peppers, dates, ginger, gulanga root, muskmelon seeds, and muscot nuts in equal quantities. Mix the nuts into olive oil. Eat 1 T. of the paste each morning before breakfast.
- Consume pills or make teas from these herbs: chickweed, sweet flag, marigold, or licorice root.
- Take 1 T. liquid lecithin daily.
- Get more lecithin by using Pam® for frying foods.
- Eat muskmelon seeds.

Other:

Poor memory often results from decreased blood flow to the brain as we mature. Studies using 120 mg/day of ginkgo biloba extract dramatically improved blood flow and memory in older adults.[46]

Menstruation (abnormal, painful)

- Keep warm. Do not lift anything heavy. Don't eat anything with vinegar, lemon, lime, or grapefruit; or rich foods like candy bars and desserts.
- Drink tea made from blue cohosh.
- Drink tea made from ½ tsp. melissa tea with ½ tsp. rue, steeped for 10 minutes, and then strained.
- Chew fennel seeds to reduce pain.
- Drink a tea made from pennyroyal daily, beginning about 2 weeks before menstruation. Pennyroyal should not be consumed if pregnant.

- One of the oldest herbal concoctions consists of: licorice, chamomile, pleurisy root, Jamaica dogwood, black cohosh, life plant, and dandelion root in an alcohol tincture. This remedy helps with both menopause and premenstrual syndrome. At one time, this remedy was sold as Lydia Pinkham's tonic.

- This is an alternative formula for tonic: goldenseal root, blessed thistle, cayenne, uva-ursi, cramp bark, false unicorn root, raspberry leaves, squaw vine, and ginger.

- To start monthly flow when there has been delayed menstruation, drink hot chamomile tea or ginger tea.

- For menstrual complaints of another nature, use tea from shave grass or horsetail grass.

- The whitish discharge from the vagina can be cleared up by administering a douche made of either 2 T. white vinegar or 2 tsp. alum per quart of lukewarm water.

Mood

Many Americans have a metabolism that is too
high in acid from alcohol, soda pop, and coffee.
Acidic people have a bitter and sour disposi-
tion.

- Reduce acidity and return metabolism to
  more normal pH by eating more vegetables.
- Take daily supplements of calcium (800 mg)
  and magnesium (800 mg).

Motion Sickness

- Take 3–4 digestive enzymes 30 minutes before the trip.

Other:

- Ginger tablets 30 minutes before the trip
help many people with motion sickness.[47]
- Employing the time-tested effectiveness of
acupressure points on the wrist. You can
purchase elastic wrist bands with a small
marble for the pressure point to relieve
problems of motion sickness. (See Appendix)

Mouth Sores

- For sore mouth from dentures, make a
cushioning poultice by soaking white lily
flowers in whisky until petals look soaked.
Use this mixture as a cushion between
gums and dentures.

- Avoid all soda, which can be irritating. Make a mouthwash using 1 tsp. each of powdered myrrh, goldenseal, and cayenne pepper blended into 1 quart water. Rinse mouth daily.
- For canker sores, drink sage tea or apply pinch of powdered sage, goldenseal powder, or raw onion.
- For chapped lips, use lanolin lotion.
- L-lysine relieves mouth sores from viral herpes.
- Apply a poultice of extract of myrrh or sage.
- At first sign of mouth sores, gargle with a mixture of 1 tsp. soda and a pinch of salt in 1 c. warm water.
- Wet the sore region, then dust with powdered goldenseal or alum.

Nerve and Sleep Disorders

- Eat light meals in the evening.
- Drink teas made from catnip, skullcap, peppermint, goldenseal, black cohosh, or blue vervain before bedtime.
- Before retiring, rub the feet well with vinegar water.
- Replace fear with strength and confidence.
- Think no evil of your neighbor. Give love and love will be returned.
- Do not exalt yourself, as pride goes before the fall.
- Consider all the nice things that people do for you and what you can do for others.
- Think good thoughts that are pure, just, and honest.

Nosebleed

- To restrain the bleeding, press the nose firmly between the finger and thumb for a few minutes.
- Place a cold wet rag on the nape of the neck for a few minutes.

Other:

- Nosebleeds can be caused by acute allergic reactions, such as from consuming milk, wheat, or other common allergenic foods.
- Use a cotton swab to apply Vicks® to the inside of the nose to prevent nosebleeds from dry winter weather.

Obesity

Temperance is the best prevention and cure. Eat less food and less often. Notice how the more a person overeats, the further nature pushes that person away from the table.

- For 3 days, consume only fresh carrot juice. This will purge the body of toxins, rest the digestive tract, and encourage rapid weight loss. You may develop a slight orange tint to the skin, which is caused by the pigment beta-carotene. It is not harmful, and will fade within a few weeks.
- Drink Chinese slim tea daily.
- Eat only raw fruit and vegetables for 3 days to get started with quick results.
- To help avoid overeating, before each meal take 2 capsules of chickweed plus 2 capsules containing: saffron, burdock, parsley, kelp, licorice, fennel, echinacea, black walnut, papaya, hawthorn berries, and mandrake.

- Eat no sweets or baked products.
- To control appetite, drink a tea prepared from 1 tsp. of orange berries from the mountain ash tree.
- For 3 days, consume only pure unsweetened grape juice.
- Up to 25% of the population are underweight. Underweight people can take 10 drops of liquid red clover extract three times daily.

Other:

- While calories do count, the most weight-inducing of calories is fat in the diet. Eat less fat and the weight will literally melt off your body.

Pain

- Mix ¼ oz. each of oil of organan, oil of hemlock, oil of lavender, oil of wintergreen, oil of
cinnamon, and oil of sassafras with 1 oz.
camphor gum and 1 quart raw dietary linseed oil. Rub this mixture externally on
burns, sores, sore throat, and other painful
areas.

- For "tennis elbow," prepare a liniment
adding 4 fresh chopped avocado seeds and 3
oz. horsetail grass to a quart of water. Cook
the water down to a pint. Add 1 pint of
rubbing alcohol and bottle the mixture.
Apply to sore area.

- For muscle soreness from long horse and
buggy trips, soak in a hot tub for 3–5 minutes. Then wrap yourself in a warm blan-
ket.

- Prepare a liniment known as "Good Samari-
tan Oil" by blending 1 quart raw linseed oil,
¼ oz. oregano oil, ½ oz. oil of sassafras, ¼

oz. wintergreen, ¼ oz. oil of lavender, and 1 oz. gum camphor. Gently rub the liniment on chest for colds.

- For back pain, mix 2 T. cayenne pepper in 1 pint cider vinegar and boil for ten minutes. Allow to cool. Apply while still warm.
- A skilled massage can relieve many forms of pain.
- Dissolve 24 aspirin tablets in 1 quart rubbing alcohol and rub liberally on sore spot.
- Apply a salve made from red tiger balm in rubbing alcohol to the sore area.
- Boil 2 T. cayenne pepper in 1 p. of cider vinegar for 10 minutes. Apply this hot solution to sore areas.
- Mix 50 aspirin, 8 grams (about ¼ oz) of wintergreen oil, and 1 pint rubbing alcohol. Rub the mixture on sore muscles or backache.
- For sciatica, the patient should lie on back, keeping knees straight. A family member should grab the ankle and raise one leg at a

time as far up over the head as possible.
Repeat 3 times. Increase repetitions and
angle of movement as pain decreases. Do
not continue if the patient finds it too painful.

- For sciatica, grip both hands on a branch or
  overhead pipe to get the entire body off the
  ground. Hang the body loosely for a few seconds to stretch the spine. Draw the knees
  up as far as possible several times then rest.

Parasites and Worms

(See a doctor first.)

- Eat hulled pumpkin seeds and follow with a
  laxative. Or cook 8 chopped pumpkin seeds
  in 1 c. boiling water and drink as a tea. For
  children, you may add 1–2 tsp. peppermint
  tea for flavor.
- Eat sauerkraut juice or garlic capsules to
  kill intestinal worms.

- Eat 3–4 dried peaches each night before retiring.
- Heat common unsalted lard to body temperature. Use a medicine dropper to place a squirt in rectum.
- Eat hot spicy chili con carne daily to purge worms.
- Keep fingernails short to avoid contaminating food.
- Entacyl® is a drug store remedy that can cure a whole family of pin worms in one day.

Pleurisy

(inflammation of the lungs)

- Take 4 capsules filled with red cayenne pepper every hour until the pain ceases. Drink plenty of water or tea afterward. Discontinue this remedy if this irritates stomach.

Pneumonia

(see a doctor first)

- Grind an onion. Add barley flour and vinegar to the onion to make a paste. Heat and spread the paste on a cloth. Apply the paste to the patient's chest.

- In a frying pan, melt 6 oz. fresh lard, 3 oz. white resin, and 3 oz. bees wax. Remove the pan from stove and blend in: 2 oz. camphor oil and 2 drams balsam Peru. Put all ingredients into a kettle and heat until melted. Strain the mixture into jars and cover. Spread the mixture on a cloth and fold the cloth over. Warm the cloth and apply this compress to the patient's chest. Cover the warm cloth with a thick flannel cloth. Keep poultice compress hot.

- Mix 2 T. lard, 2 T. flour, 1 tsp. soda, 1 tsp. black pepper, and 1 tsp. mustard. Never put a plaster made with mustard directly against the skin. Spread the mixture on cloth and lay the cloth on the patient's chest, poultice side up.

Poison Ivy and Oak

- Apply a poultice of powdered alum in Vaseline®.

- Bathe the affected parts in sassafras tea.

- Apply a poultice of crushed jewelweed stems and leaves.

- Wash affected parts with tansy tea.

- Add 2 tsp. lobelia to 1 c. boiling water. Let stand. Apply this mixture to the affected area.

-

  Soak the affected parts in a solution of Epsom salts and water for 30 minutes daily.

- Bathe the affected area with a warm solution of salt water.

- Boil a 2x4 inch section of sprig oak bark in 1 quart water for 5 minutes. Then simmer for 1 hour. Apply the liquid to the affected area for relief of itching.

- Wash skin region with tea from sassafras, jewelweed, or broom sage herbs.

- Rub the inside of a banana, lemon, or orange skin on the affected parts.

- Apply Caladryl® from the drugstore.

Poisoning

- Easiest way to treat poisoning is to induce vomiting by giving Ipecac® from the drugstore. Do not induce vomiting if patient is in convulsions or unconscious.

- Be sure to keep the number of your nearest poison control center handy by the phone. Call 911 for emergencies.

Poultice and Bone Knitter

- Make a tea from: white oak bark, comfrey root, marshmallow root, mullein, black walnut hulls, gravel root, wormwood, lobelia, and skullcap. Drink this tea daily to speed the healing of a broken bone.
- For sores and boils, apply a poultice of: ½ c. beeswax cut fine, 1 c. lard (goose is best), 1 tsp. powdered resin melted together slowly over the stove; then cooled.
- Mix 1 oz. resin, 1 oz. beeswax, and 4 oz. mutton tallow. Heat until melted. Stir in 1 dram pulverized vertergris. Allow the mixture to cool and then form it into a roll about ¾ inch in diameter. Apply this "Green Mountain Salve" to wounds.
- For a poultice that heals bruises; mix ½ lb. fresh lard, 3 oz. white resin, 2 drams balsam of Peru, ¼ lb. beeswax, and 2 oz. pulverized camphor. Melt the ingredients

slowly over low heat. Allow to cool in jars and apply to the bruise.

- Drink comfrey tea 3 times daily. At the same time, take bonemeal capsules daily.

- To draw poison out of a wound, make a poultice from ¼ c. each (lump the size of an egg) of hog's lard, beeswax, rosin, and hard brown laundry soap shaved fine. Heat ingredients slowly in an iron kettle until they dissolve. Pour into a jar and cool until hard. Apply the poultice to the wound.

- Make a poultice to draw out poisons. Mix chaparral, comfrey, red clover blossoms, pine tar, mullein, beeswax, plantain, olive oil, mutton, tallow, chickweed, and poke root. Apply this poultice to ulcers, burns, and boils.

- To help disinfect a wound, make a poultice of equal parts sulphur and alum. Sprinkle the poultice on broken skin.

- Apply a poultice of fresh crushed peach leaves to bruises.

- To help disinfect a wound, soak the sore in a mixture of 1 gallon of hot water with 3 T. hardwood ashes.

- This remedy was used to save a badly injured leg that would have been amputated. Mix 1 lb. finely pulverized resin, 1 lb. mutton tallow shaved fine, 2 oz. pure olive oil, 2 oz granulated sugar. Mix all ingredients cold—do not heat. Apply the remedy three times daily to the affected parts.

- Apply a grated vegetable—raw potato, fig, carrot, red beet, or onion—to a skin area for relief and healing.

- Mix 1 T. Epsom salt with 2 T. lard and apply to skin.

- Finely grate raw red beets. Fill a cheese-cloth bag with the gratings. Then apply the bag to the skin area.

- Mix raw egg yolk with 1 tsp. sugar and apply to lump.

- To help reduce polyps, especially in the nose region, take 2 ginseng capsules and 2–5 grams/day of vitamin C.
- Fry ½ lb. mutton tallow and strain. Hard-boil 3 dozen eggs and mash fine. Mix tallow and eggs on stove and add ½ c. olive oil, 1.5 lb. unsalted butter, 3 handfuls each of water balsam, sage, rue, and wild horseradish. Apply this mixture to cuts, burns, and sores.
- Mix one pound clover blossoms with 1 pound Vaseline® and heat in the hot sun or in the oven for 1 hour. Strain through cheesecloth and store in jar. Apply to chapped hands and teats.

Pregnancy

Amish women tend to look on the facets of pregnancy as a normal occurrence, rather than a burden.

- Avoid pennyroyal if you want to get pregnant. Pennyroyal discourages conception.

- To calm stress in a pregnant woman, use a tea made from black cohosh, cayenne, hops flowers, mistletoe, lobelia, skullcap, wood betany, valerian root, and lady's slipper.

- If labor is overdue and the baby is ready to come, consume 1 c. of blue cohosh tea followed by 1 c. of squaw vine tea.

- A minor complaint of pregnancy is kidney trouble (or edema, fluid retention), which Amish women remedy with diuretic teas like sweet fennel, watermelon seeds, parsley, or bearberry.

- Most Amish women take an herbal mixture throughout pregnancy. They take 1–3 capsules of: equal parts of red raspberry and squaw vine daily. Others use loose tea, since it is cheaper.

- For the last 6 weeks of pregnancy, use an herbal mixture of: squaw vine, blessed thistle, black cohosh, false unicorn, red raspberry leaves, and lobelia. Normal dosage is 1–2 capsules/3 times daily. Amish women claim that this herbal remedy helps promote faster and easier delivery by providing elasticity to the pelvic and vaginal areas.

- Another formula which helps both mother and infant is horsetail grass, oat straw, comfrey, and lobelia.
- To stop post-partum (after birth) hemorrhaging, take the herbs, ergot or shepherd's purse.
- To reverse thinning hair after delivery, take 20 drops daily of red clover tops tincture.

Miscarriage:

- To help avoid miscarriage, drink tea from ½ handful of red raspberry leaves in 1 c. of boiling water.
- To help avoid miscarriage, drink tea from false unicorn, goldenseal root, squaw vine, and orange peel.

Morning Sickness and Nausea:

- Eat 2 T. brewer's yeast, extra iron, bone meal, and vitamin E daily.

- To stop nausea, drink a tea made from one (only one!!) peach leaf.

- Drink red raspberry tea.

- Eat a few soda crackers about 15 minutes before getting out of bed. Eat a small amount of crackers several times through-out the day to settle the stomach.

- Eat one cup of yogurt in the evening before retiring.

- For the nausea or morning sickness of pregnancy, drink a tea made from red rasp-berry, spearmint leaf, alfalfa leaf, lemon verbena, lemon balm, nettle leaf, fennel seed, lemon grass leaf, and stevia leaf.

Lactation:

- To encourage milk supply, mother should drink 1 quart of catnip tea daily. This calms both mother and infant.

- Marshmallow, blessed thistle, or alfalfa tea help with mother's milk supply.
- For improved milk output, eat oatmeal gruel three times daily.
- For improved milk output, drink a tea from: fennel seeds, spearmint leaf, coriander seeds, lemon verbena, anise seed, chamomile flower, borage tops, blessed thistle leaf, althea root, lemon grass leaf, stevia leaf, and fenugreek seed.

Breast Lumps:

- Make a poultice from equal parts of wintergreen oil, olive, and spirits of turpentine (not same as commercial type). Do not use while pregnant or nursing.
- Make a poultice from equal parts of castor oil and oil of wintergreen (genuine, not synthetic). Do not use while pregnant or nursing.
- Avoid eating chocolate.

Other:

- Active pregnant women usually have an easier delivery than women who are sedentary and get overweight.

Prostate

- Drink tea from burdock (gletta).
- Drink strong peppermint tea every hour.
- Take an enema of warm water, coffee, or salt water.
- Make a tea daily from the silk of 6 ears of corn, boiled and then steeped for 10 minutes. Drink 1 c. of this tea three times daily. This remedy also acts as a diuretic.
- Chew fresh roasted pumpkin seeds. This remedy also acts as worm-killer (vermifuge). As an option, take tablets of pumpkin seed oil.
- Tea from Pau d'Arco helps.
- Take 50–100 mg zinc supplements daily.

Other:

- Herbs of saw palmetto (serenoa repens) have been clinically proven to reduce swollen prostate gland in humans.[48]

Rheumatic Fever

- Take pure mixed natural vitamin E before breakfast each day.

Rheumatism and Arthritis

- Make an herbal tonic. Cut up 6 oranges, 6 lemons, 6 grapefruit. Cook the sliced fruit (peels and all) in 2 quarts of water and strain. Then add ½ c. Epsom salt. Let the water cook down to 1 quart and let stand overnight. Take 1 T. 3 times daily.
- Do not eat sugar, pork, or strawberries.
- These problems can be caused by food poisoning from nightshade family. Avoid egg plant, green peppers, tomatoes, and pota-

toes, which contain substances that are harmful to sensitive individuals.

- Make an herbal preparation from yucca, comfrey root, chaparral, alfalfa, burdock root, buckthorn bark, black cohosh root, parsley, slippery elm bark, yarrow, chelated trace minerals, cayenne, and lobelia.
- Take capsules of Devil's claw leaves.
- Drink 3 oz. pure aloe vera juice 3 times daily.
- Reduce fat in the diet to clear up back pain. Eat less eggs, beef, pork, and cheese.
- Take extra calcium as a supplement.
- Consume extra vitamin C (1–5 grams).
- Apply a poultice of equal parts olive oil and ammonia.
- Mix 2 oz. wintergreen oil with 1 pint rubbing alcohol. Rub the mixture along the spine.
- Make tea from ½ oz. each of burdock, dock root, sassafras bark, dandelion, and dwarf elder in 2 quarts of water. Boil down to 1

quart. Take 2 T.
3 times daily.

- Mix the juice of 3 lemons with 1 pint cold water, ¼ c. Epsom salts, and a pinch cream of tartar. Take 2 tsp. first thing in morning.

- Eat 5 pokeberries daily following this procedure to begin. Eat one pokeberry on the first day. Eat two pokeberries on the second, and so on till reaching 5 berries daily.

- Gather 3 oz. olive oil, 2 oz. charcoal, 1 lb. figs, 1.5 lb. raisins, 1 oz. glycerine, 3 oz. powdered senna, and 1 oz. slippery elm powder. Grind the fruit. Mix in the dry ingredients. Next add the oil and glycerine. Mix with hands and form into walnut size balls. Eat one ball in morning and one in evening for first week. After the first week, take only one ball in the evening and none in morning.

- Include 4–10 bonemeal tablets as part of the daily diet, especially for back pain.

- Pour 1 quart boiling water over 6 T. alfalfa seeds and steep for 15 minutes. Drink 2 cups daily—morning and evening. Begin with only ½ c. twice daily.

- Take 1 tsp. cod liver oil daily, washed down with unsweetened fruit juice.

- Drink goat's milk.

- Prepare a mixture of 6 lemons squeezed and cut up, 1 pint alfalfa honey, 1 small can cream of tartar, 1 tsp. Epsom salts in 1 quart boiling water. Let stand overnight. Strain and keep refrigerated. Take 1 T. in morning and another T. at night.

- Eat one boiled lemon each day for 50 days.

- Mix 1 tsp. cider vinegar in 1 glass tomato juice and drink 2 or more glasses daily, preferably before meals (on an empty stomach).

- Dissolve ½ tsp. Epsom salts in 2 cups water which has been boiled and cooled. Add the juice of 2 lemons to the water. Then pour the liquid into a glass jar and keep refrigerated. Take 2 T. each morning before breakfast. Aspirin along with this remedy may help ease pain.

- Take 50–100 mg. zinc daily.
- If symptoms are actually from gout, abstain from red meat.
- Mix 1 pint gin, 2 oz. juniper berries, 1 T. Epsom salts, and 1 T. sugar. Take 1 tsp. of the mixture 3 times daily.
- Pack a quart can with ferns. Fill the can with rubbing alcohol and set in it sun for 4 weeks. Rub this lotion on ailing parts.

Ringworm

- Apply a poultice of 2 parts lard and 1 part sulphur to the affected area. Wear old clothes when using , because this poultice will soil clothes.
- Hold an ice pack to the sore for 5–10 minutes.

- Wash the area or hair with tar soap and borax. Then moisten the spots with a solution made from ½ tsp. goldenseal, ½ tsp. myrrh, and 1 tsp. bloodroot and steeped in a pint of boiling water.
- Drink at least 1 c. goldenseal tea daily.

Sexual Desire

- Chew on ginseng root daily.
- An herbal combination used often by the Amish for men over 40 includes Damiana, Siberian ginseng, echinacea, Fo-Ti, Gotu-Kola, sarsaparilla, and saw palmetto.

Other:

- Married men live 5 years longer than bachelors. Men who kiss their wives daily live an average of 5 years longer than married men who do not regularly kiss their wives. British widowers have a 40% higher heart attack death rate than their married peers.
- Thyroid. It is estimated that 40% or more of the population suffers from low thyroid output (hypothyroidism), especially as we age. Low thyroid can influence many processes, including sex drive [49]

Recommendation: If your basal temperature first thing in the morning is below 97.8 F, you are a likely candidate for thyroid supplementation. Work with your doctor, since thyroid supplements are a prescription medication. As an option, you can stimulate the thyroid gland by providing the proper raw ingredients for its functioning, including iodine (10 drops liquid kelp) and 15 drops of thyroid stimulant from Natural Herbal Extract (See Appendix).

Shingles

- Shingles may be caused by nervousness; so consume more B vitamins and nerve tonic teas.
- Take up to 6 grams daily of L-lysine.
- Apply a hot cloth soaked in a solution of pine bark and mulberry leaves.

Sinus Congestion

(See also the section on Colds.)

- See the section on Allergies for information on a nasal purge with salt water.
- To relieve sinus congestion of colds and flu, add peppermint or spearmint oil to a bedroom vaporizer at night.
- Place a pinch of goldenseal on the tongue.
- Drink goldenseal tea while eliminating all dairy products from the diet.
- Mix a handful of pennyroyal leaves in 6 oz. sweet almond oil until the oil turns green. Then add a few grams of horehound powder. Use a few drops of this mixture in the nose for decongestion.
- To cut down the bacteria count in the air, use pine, cedar, or mint oil in a vaporizer. Europeans have long known that a sanitarium in an evergreen forest is more conducive to recuperation. Some hospitals bring

potted pine trees into the rooms to help patients recover.

- Use the Olbas inhaler from Switzerland, containing oils of menthol, peppermint, and eucalyptol..

- Rub the outside of the nose area with Vicks® before retiring at night.

- Mix 1 quart water, ¼ c. vinegar, and 2 T. honey. Drink 1 c. of this mixture daily.

- Use an eye dropper to apply a small amount of warm mineral oil (baby oil) in the nose. While applying hand head over the bed to keep oil inside the nose.

- Mix 2 c. water and 2 T. vinegar in a kettle and boil. Put a towel over your head and around the kettle in order to inhale the steam. Do this for 5–10 minutes daily.

- Mix 1 c. warm water, ¼ tsp. salt, ¼ tsp. Listerine®. Use as a nasal purge as described in the section on Allergies.

- Drink tea or chew sections from angelica root.

- Mix 1 pint water, 1 tsp. salt, 1 tsp. peppermint oil, 1 tsp. boric acid, 1 tsp. baking soda and use as nasal purge as described in the section on Allergies.
- Drink tea from mullein.

Other:

Although many Americans take antibiotics for a cold, antibiotics do nothing for a viral infection and may reduce the immune system's ability to fight the cold. Take medication only when it is absolutely necessary.

Sprains

- Immediately after the injury, apply cold towels to the site (to reduce swelling). The next day, alternate between cold and hot applications. On the third day, use hot towels (to improve healing).
- Apply a hot poultice of vinegar.

- Fry black root in lard and cool. Rub the cooled lard on the sprained part.
- Drink boneset tea.

Spurs

- Take supplements of calcium and magnesium (800 mg. each).
- Wear good arch supports in your shoes.

Stomach Problems

- Eat an occasional soda cracker.
- Every morning before breakfast, drink a glass of hot water with 2 tsp. cider vinegar and 2 tsp. honey.
- Chew caraway seeds for an upset stomach.
- Each morning, drink a tea made from ¼ tsp. sage or goldenseal in 1 c. hot water.
- Mix "go back" drops by combining 1 oz. glycerine, 10 drops aconite tincture, and 1

oz. rain water. Take 3–5 drops twice daily for 3 days. Wait 3 days and repeat dose.

- For heartburn, drink ¼ c. water with ¼ tsp. baking soda.
- Drink tea from burdock root.
- For pain in stomach, be aware of foods that may cause an allergy.
- Drink a tea made from goldenseal one hour before mealtime. Other helpful teas for stomach problems include teas made from thyme, cayenne, fennel, ginseng, sage, sassafras, slippery elm, and chickweed.
- For a stomach ulcer, consume 2 T. sauerkraut juice before eating.
- Mix 1 T. mutton tallow in a ½ c. of hot milk taken 30 minutes before mealtime. Follow the milk with by a glass of cold water.
- To build stomach muscles and get rid of bulging stomach, lie flat on the back on a padded floor. Raise both feet slowly as high as is comfortable, , keeping knees straight. Then lower legs almost to the floor and re-

peat this exercise. Start this exercise slowly with 4–5 repetitions, then build up to higher repetitions.

Stroke

- To help encourage recovery in the damaged tissue, use physical therapy and bathe the affected body parts with tea made from cayenne pepper and water.

Sweaty Feet

- Wear white cotton stockings.
- Bathe feet frequently.
- For feet that do not sweat, walk through morning dew in bare feet, then rub feet vigorously with towel.
- To squelch foot odor, sprinkle baking soda powder inside shoes.
- For tired feet, soak feet for 20 minutes in solution of 1 quart hot water with 1 tsp. boric acid.

Throat

- For dry throat common in speakers, chew small pieces of dried calamus root.
- Chew a piece of ginseng root.
- Take 1 tsp. Olba's Oil, found in health food stores.
- For strep throat, apply a poultice of grated garden beets on the outside of the throat. Freshen the poultice when the beets turn a greenish color. Continue changing and applying this poultice until the beets do not change color.
- Suck on fresh cloves of garlic.
- Take 10 drops of red clover tops 2–3 times daily.
- For swollen throat glands, gargle with a mixture made from 7 lime rinds boiled in milk.
- For swollen glands, apply a piece of flannel soaked in warm vinegar. Do not squeeze glands!!

- Drink tea from mullein and lobelia.
- For hoarseness, beat stiff the white of a fresh egg. Add juice of one lemon, 1 T. glycerine, 1 tsp. sugar. Take a swallow often until hoarseness disappears.
- For tonsillitis, gargle with tea made from red clover tops. Externally apply a poultice of onions. Or take thymus extract, available from a health food store. You also can make an herbal preparation from equal parts skullcap, lobelia, valerian root, myrrh, gum, black cohosh, and cayenne.

Tobacco Habit (To Quit)

- For several days, drink only unsweetened fruit and vegetable juices to cleanse the system.
- Take a relaxing hot bath each day.
- Drink tea from red clover for cleansing.
- Drink tea from gentian, magnolia, or catnip to reduce cravings.

Tonic (Purifier, Energizer, Toner)

- Boil down ½ oz. of Snake Root (Aristolochia serpentaria) in a pint of boiling water for 2 hours. Take 1 tsp. three times daily.
- Eat watercress, alfalfa sprouts, or dandelion leaves in a salad.
- Make homemade ginger ale by chopping up a fresh ginger root in a quart of water. Simmer until water is yellow, strain, add honey and carbonated water.
- Soak 3 quarts of dandelion flowers in 2 quarts of water for 3 days. Strain and add 2 pounds sugar, 1 sliced lemon, and 1 T. yeast. Let the mixture stand for 4 days and bottle it. Use 1 T. before each meal.
- Take 2 oz. each of sarsaparilla root, sassafras root, spikenard root, black birch bark, yellow dock root, and spruce needles. Boil ingredients in 4 gallons of water for 25 minutes, strain, and let cool. Add 1 lb.

brown sugar and 3 T. yeast and let it ferment (allow an escape valve for gases). Bottle after 3 days. Drink 1 c. as needed.

- Use a leather glove to pick fresh stinging nettles. Boil 1 oz. of stinging nettles in 1 pint of water and take 1 T. of the liquid daily.

Tonsillitis

- Mix 1 T. yellow root, ½ tsp. salt, 1 tsp. garden sage, and ½ tsp. soda. Simmer the ingredients in 1 c. water for 30 minutes. Then cool and add ½ c. cider vinegar. Gargle every few hours with this solution.
- Swab the tonsils with a cotton swab dipped in a mixture of ½ oz. iodine and ½ oz. glycerine.
- Mix 1 T. yellow dock root, 1 tsp. garden sage, ½ tsp. salt, and ½ tsp. soda in 1 c. water. Cool the liquid and add ½ c. cider vinegar. Gargle with this solution every 3 hours.

- At first sign of oncoming sore throat, take 1 tsp. of honey every hour.
- Sip the juice of 1 lemon mixed with 1 tsp. honey. This remedy may be added to hot water to make a tea mixture.
- Put a peeled and cleaned garlic bulb in the mouth and bite on it regularly. Discomfort will lessen.
- Make a gargle solution using 4 oz water, ½ tsp. salt and ½ tsp. soda.
- Make a gargle solution with 1 c. hot water, 1 tsp. vinegar, and sprinkling of hot pepper powder. Gargle every 15 minutes.

Toothache and Teeth

Sugar is expensive: you pay for it twice; once at the grocery store and again at the dentist.

- Cut down on dental bills by adding bone-meal and wheat germ to baked bread and cookies. Both help build strong teeth.

- Eat asparagus (fresh or canned) everyday and you will either have no problems, or be able to bear the pain until you can get to a dentist.
- Soak cotton in oil of clove and place the cotton next to sore tooth.
- Cut a fresh fig in half and lay it next to sore tooth.
- Drink tea made from equal parts of horse-tail grass, comfrey root, oat straw, and lobelia.
- Fry an onion until it is hot. Then pour the onion into a small cloth bag. If the toothache is on the right side of the mouth, place the bag on the pulse of the right wrist region. If the toothache is on the left side of the mouth, place the bag on the pulse of the left wrist region.
- Place ice on the sore tooth.
- Fill the tooth cavity with a small cotton plug soaked in cayenne, peppermint oil, and aspirin.

Ulcer and Colitis

- Drink 6 oz of cabbage juice a ½ hour before meals. Prepare the juice by blending 3 cups of chopped cabbage with 16 oz water in a blender. Strain before drinking.
- Take capsules of comfrey and fenugreek.
- Take capsules of combing slippery elm, comfrey root, lobelia, ginger, and wild yam.
- Eat a bit of cabbage with each meal. Chew the cabbage slowly.
- Drink goldenseal tea.
- Consume only grapes or grape juice for 3 days. A person must be in good health to attempt this fast.
- Drink glass of aloe vera daily.

Varicose Veins

- Drink 3 cups daily of white oak bark tea.
- To strengthen the muscles and blood vessels in the leg region, jump rope daily. Be-

gin this exercise regimen slowly. Jump 1 minute per session and build up to 5 minutes.

- Eat plenty of fresh garlic and take vitamin E supplements.
- To relieve the pain of varicose veins, bathe the legs in vinegar 3 times daily.
- For ulcers that form on varicose veins, apply dry powdered sugar.

Vinegar

Vinegar has so many uses. Because it is so inexpensive and non-toxic, vinegar merits its own section.

- Use vinegar for underarm deodorant after bathing.
- Use vinegar diluted in a glass of warm water as a gargle for sore throat.
- Soak soiled clothes in vinegar to remove stubborn stains.
- Rub vinegar on insect stings.
- Use vinegar as hair rinse.
- Rinse diapers in vinegar to help prevent diaper rash.
- When soaking in hot water, rinse with vinegar for a cooling sensation.
- Boil vinegar in pot on stove and inhale vapors to clear plugged sinuses.
- To help prevent food poisoning when visiting foreign countries or questionable res-

taurants, take 1 T. vinegar in a glass of water 30 minutes before eating.

Warts

- Soak a bandage in castor oil and tie the bandage around the wart region.
- Apply celandine or milkweed juice.
- Touch the wart with a toothpick soaked in castor oil. This remedy also helps eliminate corns.
- Rub wart with raw potato peelings.
- Wash wart region 3 times daily with baking soda and water solution.
- Apply the milky juice of a dandelion to the wart.
- Rub the wart each day with a piece of white chalk.
- Apply the juice from milkweed to the wart.
- Apply wood ashes to the wart.
- Apply iodine daily.
- Rub garlic on wart daily.

Afterword

Who Are the Amish?

The Amish were born from the religious turmoil of the Ana-Baptist movement in 16th Century Switzerland. In 1525, they started their own church with their own beliefs, which included separation of church and state and adult baptism. They believed that children who were baptized knew little of true faith and merely gave lip service to their religion. The word *Amish* comes from Jakob Ammann, an influential leader from the new church.

Very soon the state church banned the new faith which began a very bloody battle of repression and extermination. The new religion was called, *Ana-Baptist,* a word which in the

Christian world at that time meant heathen or devil worshippers. Many of these early Amish faced the bonfire, garroting or beheading. Terrible tortures were committed on the Amish who would not retract their faith.

The Martyr's Mirror, a book that records in detail how many of these early Christians were tortured, was published in 1660. Today this book, along with the Bible and the Ausbund, one of the oldest Protestant hymnals, are the three most important books in any Amish household.

By 1711, the Swiss government had had enough of the Ana-Baptists and many were loaded on ships and sent to Holland, leaving all their possessions behind. Starting all over, they scattered throughout central Europe to Germany, France, and Russia. But it was only when they began migrating to America sometime after 1700, that the Amish began to grow and prosper.

At first the Amish feared migrating to American because of the long and dangerous ocean voyage. However, their journey to America was to be their survival. The American Constitution guaranteed freedom of religion for all. And there was land, plenty of it, and it was cheap. They could only rent land in Europe, so the dream of owning their own land was like a miracle. On October 8, 1737, the ship, *Charming Nancy*, arrived in Philadelphia with the first group of Amish. Most moved west where they settled in Ohio, Pennsylvania, Indiana, Illinois, Iowa, and Nebraska. Today Amish people live in at least twenty states and in Canada. Ohio has more Amish than any other state, followed by Pennsylvania and Indiana.

Many of these groups follow slightly different traditions. For example, some ride in gray buggies, some in black buggies, and others in white and in yellow buggies. Some dress codes are a little different as well, but their basic beliefs clearly set them apart as Amish.

What the Land Means to the Amish

The Amishman loves the land. Next to the Bible, the land is the most important thing in his life. He believes it is a gift from God and that man must care for the land with every ounce of his strength. And certainly the Amish do carefully and tediously take care of their land. Farming has become one of the tenets of the Amish religion. Over the years they have developed an acute farm sense. Some of the most modern techniques in farming were introduced by the Amish long before they were used elsewhere.

Many Amish farms have been in the family for more than 200 years. They are handed down from father to son, generation after generation. The Amish consider their rural way of life essential to living separate from the world.

What is *Old of the Good?*

The Amish will accept some progress but will not let it destroy their community life. They carefully choose inventions and machines based on how they will affect their lives. They see nothing inconsistent about writing with a magic marker and driving a horse and carriage. While telephones are forbidden in their homes, they are permitted to use a pay phone. But the use of electricity is another matter. The Amish feel that plugging into an electrical socket will change their whole way of thinking and their bond with nature. The conveniences that electricity could provide would destroy simplicity, humility, and communal dependence.

The Amish *Home Sweet Home*

The Amish Home is usually wood frame and painted white. It has a solid no-nonsense feel

about it. Often, in addition to the main structure there may be a summer kitchen and a
wash house. Many have porches with the traditional porch swing, the perfect place for a
courting couple to spend the evening. Although
the Amish home is somewhat plain, great
beauty is seen in the beds of brilliantly colored
geraniums, marigolds, nasturtiums, and other
flowers which decorate yards from spring to
autumn. Carefully-tended vegetable gardens
are lush with bright tomatoes, cucumbers,
squash, corn, pumpkins, and peppers.

Amish orchards also provide fruit to last
through the cold season. The Amish family
who does not have fruit trees will help a neighbor gather his bounty and take payment in
fruit. In the fall, much of summer's harvest is
canned or stored in root cellars for the long
winters.

In early winter, the Amish butcher their hogs,
often one for each family member. The entire

family helps in preparing the hams, pork chops, and bacon and in chopping the leftovers for delicious Amish sausage and puddings. Some say their hams, which are sugar-cured an seasoned with good old hickory smoke flavor are the best in the world.

Amish homes and barns do not have lightning rods because the believe that if lightning strikes, it is the will of God. If lightning burns a house or barn to the ground, the people of the church help rebuild it. And although the Amish do not carry insurance, when hardship occurs, they can receive assistance from "Amish Aid," a fund each family contributes to for such emergencies. Also, friends and relatives give personal possessions to a family in trouble.

The Kitchen Is the Center
for Amish Family Life

In many Amish homes, the coal and wood burning stove in the kitchen is the only source of heat. So, the family gathers in the kitchen for warmth as well as companionship. The kitchen table is where everybody eats. Dishes are plain heavy china and utensils are usually stainless steel, never silver. Off the kitchen is the pantry always filled with enough to generously feed company dropping in.

The Amish women spend a great deal of their time in the kitchen cooking, baking, and canning. Today Amish cookbooks are available in many bookstores with the traditional Amish recipes like shoofly pie, chow-chow, noodles, chocolate cake, hearty soups, jellies, and jams.

An Amish woman's day has little time for back fence gossiping. Not only does she make her own clothes, but work clothes for the men in the family and all of the children's clothing. She acts as a barber, doctor, and even carpenter, often mending and fixing the house. On Monday mornings, clotheslines stretch over every yard loaded with clean clothes flapping in the wind. And she does all this in an old-fashioned wringer washer sometimes equipped with a gasoline engine. And most Amish homes till have the old-style, solid-metal sad irons which are heated on stoves for necessary ironing.

Staying Healthy with Old-Time Remedies

The Amish housewife keeps a close watch to see that every member of the family has a good appetite, sleeps well, and is strong and active. At the first sign of any illness, she goes to her medicine cabinet stocked with home remedies for colds, upset stomach, sore throat, sleeplessness, backache, headache, and even special tonics that renew vigor. The remedies are made from formulas passed by word of mouth from one generation to another.

Many of the ingredients for these remedies come from the Amish woman's carefully tended herb garden. Every garden grows a variety of teas, such as catnip, peppermint, sassafras, sage, and others. There are also plenty of parsley, garlic, chives, and other medicinal herbs to keep the family healthy and fit.

Speaking of these home remedies, one Amish woman was quoted as saying, *A doctor was usually called as a last resort, after everything else failed, and this wasn't often.*

How Do the Amish Relax and Have Fun?

It is a mistake to think that there is not a lot of happiness in the Amish home. If the Amish work together, they also play together. There are quilting bees, apple-paring parties, auctions, town trips, visits, reunions, barn raisings, church Sundays, and loads of weddings. And Amish women even enjoy a game of baseball or Frisbee.

When chores are finished, Amish children have plenty of time for fun and games. The boys love baseball and play with spirit from spring until the snow flies. The girls enjoy games all girls do—jump rope, hide-and-seek, and chasing through the grassy fields. Cold weather and snow brings fun for everyone—ice skating, sledding, snowball fights, and horse-drawn sleigh rides over the snowy hills to visit friends and relatives. Although this simple way of life may seem like all work and no play, it is far from it.

Sunday *Go to Meeting*

Sunday is very much the Lord's Day among the Amish and all work ceases. Their preaching services are held every other Sunday and may last as long as three hours. Families living within a district take turns having services in their homes. Driving through Amish country on a Sunday, you can see as many as forty to fifty buggies parked in a yard for services.

There is much preparation for this special day. Stables must be cleaned and yards cut and trimmed, walls are painted and fences whitewashed. The meeting benches must be brought in and set up. Often on Saturday before preaching, more than a dozen women will gather to bake breads and pies and to be sure there's plenty of coffee, pickles, red beets, and jams for the meal after the service. Everyone enjoys this social time after the preaching on Sunday. Discussions range from happenings of the day, crops, and children to world events.

The Amish keep up with what's going on in the world and speak intelligently on a variety of subjects. Some of their information comes from the most widely read Amish newspaper, *The Budget,* published in Sugarcreek, Ohio. It circulates to more than thirty states.

Amish preachers are chosen for life and receive not special training or salary. In fact, every Amishman is
expected to be ready to accept the call from God if it comes to him. Amish bishops are the ones who administer discipline, but major decisions are made by the vote of each church member.

The Amish Tongue

The Amish speak in three distinctive languages. First, all Amish in the United States speak the Pennsylvania Dutch language. This language is not a degenerate form of German but a dialect of High German that is still spoken in the Rhineland area of Germany today. They also use English when speaking to non-Amish people. An Amish person will switch from the dialect to English when it is more comfortable for the occasion and often you will hear both languages being spoken at one table. Their third language is High German. This is used for worship services, Bible reading, praying, and singing hymns.

The Amish Simple Way of Dress

The Amish have retained dress styles common in Europe during the seventeenth and eighteenth centuries. Though there have been some gradual changes, they have not adopted the styles and fashions of other Americans.

Like their mothers and grandmothers, girls wear long dresses about eight inches from the floor. Dresses of little girls are often bright colors, such as teal, royal blue, green, and purple. They do not wear plaids, prints, or polka dots— only plain colors. Up to eight years old, girls wear a pinafore called a *Schlupp Schotzli*, over their dresses. Older girls wear aprons and capes fastened with straight pins. Some of the older girls wear white prayer caps like their mothers as well as black stockings and shoes that tie. The Amish women never wear jewelry, make-up, lipstick, or perfume, and they do not cut their hair. They rarely wear red since many consider that it stands for the devil and lust.

Amish men and boys wear plain-colored shirts and paints with no hip pockets, cuffs, or zippers. In place of a fly, there is a large flap that hooks on both sides. A special kind of coat with a split tail must always be worn for church and most Amish men and boys can still be seen wearing the plain black, wide-brimmed hat. A beard is required of all adult male members of the church. Boys are clean-shaven until they marry. At that time, they begin to grow a beard, but mustaches are forbidden.

Family Means Everything to the Amish

When the Amish speak of family they're talking about a mother, father, and six, seven, eight—even ten—child-ren or more. And quite often even grandmothers and grandfathers live in the same house sharing the responsibilities and the joy of family life. The Amish do not permit divorce and separation is practically unknown.

Amish families are very much like the big family of
the last century. In the winter, they gather

around the kitchen stove eating popcorn while the mother knits, the children play games, and the father reads from
the German Bible. The Amish father teaches non-aggression and non-competition. He believes that it's the enjoyment of the game that counts.

In the typical Amish family, everyone is instructed to do his or her job in the best possible way. Amish children begin to assist their parents at four or five years old. As children master one task, bigger ones are given. Young Amish boys are introduced to all aspects of the farm operation at an early age and eventually will do the major part of the heavy farm work.

The girls take care of the younger children and begin to cook, bake, garden, and sew along with their mothers. They are preparing for the most important things in life—motherhood and being a good farm wife. Nothing pleases the Amish parent more than seeing their children grow up to be honest, hard-working, and thrifty.

Because the Amish home is one of the most stable in the world, the Amish child is less likely to get into serious trouble. Every child is greatly loved and receives plenty of attention from parents as well as numerous brothers, sisters, and scores of relative. The Amish child may not have a great many material possessions, but he always has the certainty that he is loved and that the large family and his church will always be behind him as long as he upholds his faith.

Reading, Writing, and Arithmetic

In 1972 the Supreme Court ruled that states could not force the Amish to send their children to public schools. Because the Amish do not believe in further education, the law requires Amish children to attend school only through the eighth grade. The Amish believe that too much education makes children too "worldly" with desires for the materialistic things they see around them. True education, according to the Amish, is the cultivation of humility, simple living, and resignation to the will of God.

The typical Amish one-room schoolhouse is from another century with its bell and pot-bellied stove. And although most Amish homes have bathrooms, there are none in the schools. Instead, two outhouses stand at an appropriate distance from the school house.

Children in grades one through eight attend school together where they learn reading, writing, and arithmetic. They also have advanced classes in German so that they can read their Bible. Unlike public school teachers, the Amish teacher did not go to college. After completing eighth grade, a good student may simply be asked to be a teacher.

The school supports the values taught in the family and helps the child to becomes a part of his or her community and to stay within it. Students do not pledge allegiance to the flag in school because the Amish do not believe in submitting to any government. When school is over for the day, the children walk home where they finish their chores and prepare for supper and a quiet evening around the kitchen stove.

A-Courting We Will Go

When Amish young people are about 16, they begin to attend Sunday night "singings." Often first dates are
arranged after these social occasions. The Amish call dating "running around." Although there is much secrecy about Amish courting, it is known that when a couple begins to go steady, he will visit her home on Saturday nights. he patiently waits until her family is sleeping, then turns a flashlight on her win-

dow. This is her signal that her date has arrived.

Their date is spent in the sitting room or the bed room, where they practice *bundling*. Bundling is an Amish custom where young couples sleep or lie together on the same bed without undressing. This old custom has its roots in Oriental as well as European tradition.

Still Traveling by Horse and Buggy

The Amish still use the horse and buggy to get around, not because they think that the automobile is evil, but because they believe that the life style the automobile brings with it will break down the family unit and the basic structure of their community. The obvious limitations of the horse and buggy assure that life is spent largely in the family and community, rather than outside of them.

Buggy design and color will vary from community to community. But a two-seated top buggy is strictly for the family. The one-seated topless buggy is preferred by the young man of courting age and he may add such luxuries as signal lights, dimmer switches and a hat rack.

All around the Amish community you will find signs of the horse—hitch rails, stores selling horse blankets and other necessary horse equipment. And no community is complete without its blacksmith shop and harness and buggy makers. The horse is greatly valued for its many functions. It not only provides transportation and power for running farm machinery but it fertilizes the fields as well.

Can the Amish Way of Life Survive?

For more than two centuries, the Amish have resisted change. But changes are quickly slipping into their simple world. For example, even the moderate use of the telephone is change.

Can this lead to a desire for other modern conveniences, particularly by the younger people? Without a doubt, technology is causing the Amish much concern as to how to hold on to their members.

So, perhaps, they won't go on without some reformation—the tractor may replace the horse—homes may one day have electricity. But these strong, resilient people have been "survivors" for hundreds of years. Though their way of life may undergo some change, their attachment to the land and devotion to the Bible will preserve the Amish people.

Apppendix A—Sources

Where to Buy Ingredients

Herbs and Vitamins

- Herbal Healer Academy
  HC 32, Box 97-B, Mt.View, AR 72560
  ph. 501-269-4177, fax 501-269-5424
  (vast herb inventory)
- Planetary Formulas
  Box 533W, Soquel, CA 95073
  ph 800-776-7701
  (herbs)
- Frontier Co.-operative
  Box 299, Norway, IA 52318
  ph.800-669-3275
  (herbs)

- Time Honored Herbs
  7217 Gulf Blvd., St. Petersburg, FL 33706
  ph.800-336-9636
- New Moon Extracts
  Box 1947, Brattleboro, VT 05301
  ph. 800-543-7279
  (herbal extracts)
- Enzymatic Therapy
  825 Challenger Dr., Greenbay, WI 54304
  ph.800-558-7372
  (herbs and vitamins)
- Vitamin Research Products
  3579 Hwy. 50 East
  Carson City, NV 89701
  ph. 800-877-2447
  (extensive line of vitamins,
  minerals, and amino acids)
- Bronson Pharmaceuticals
  1945 Craig Rd.
  St. Louis, MO 63146
  ph. 800-235-3200
  (vitamins)

- Min Tong
  3252 Ramona St.
  Richmond, CA 94564
  ph. 800-538-1333
  (herbs)

Easy to Take Powder Vitamin C

- Seraphim
  800-525-7372

Cranberry Extract Pills

- Ecological Formulas
  1061 Shary Circle
  Concord, CA, 94518
  ph. 800-888-4585

Special Natural Vitamin E

- A.C. Grace Company
  1100 Quitman Rd.
  Big Sandy, TX 75755
  ph. 903-636-4368

Special Mixture of EPA (fish oil) and GLA (borage oil)

- Eicotek, Inc.
  21 Tioga Way
  Marblehead, MA 01945
  ph. 800-233-3426

Aloe Vera with Active Ingredient

- Royal Body Care
  10575 Newkirk
  Dallas, TX 75220
  ph. 214-401-0052

Salve for Sun Spots on Skin

- Cansema, Applied Botanical Research
  Box 350
  Lake Charles, LA 70602-0350
  ph. 800-256-2253

Wrist Band to Relieve Motion Sickness

- Solutions
  Box 6878
  Portland, OR 97228
  ph.800-342-9988

Amish Life and Christian Education Materials

- Basic Christian Education
  Box D
  Nottawa, MI 49075

Appendix B—Healthy Lifestyle

What Is a Healthy Lifestyle?

Many of the recommendations listed in this book assume that the person is already living a healthy lifestyle, as the Amish do, and has eliminated most possible causative factors for their symptoms. Not only is the "healthy lifestyle" not taught in American schools, but we are continuously bombarded with commercials for expensive junk food and drink. Even physicians are woefully unprepared on the subject of nutrition and healthy lifestyle.

This section is included for a good reason—you can take the home remedies recommended in the earlier part of this book, but if you are obese, sedentary, stressed, smoking, drinking, and doing other major wrongs, then a little herb tea will be unable to reverse the negative forces of your lifestyle. It is crucial that you follow the recommendations in this section PLUS do whatever the book recommends for your symptoms.

I have found it unwise to lay out a detailed food and exercise program for people. By the second day, patients are out of a food, or eat at an aunt's house, discarding the program altogether. However, when you become your own nutritionist, you can take good judgment into any unforeseen circumstances and make good decisions.

Navigational school for sailors does not include an escort around the world to show people how to find everything. Instead, sailors are taught how to use a sextant, compass, and map. From those tools trained sailors can find their way anywhere, because they have what they need to support good judgment. Similarly, I cannot follow you around for the rest of your life, tell-

ing you what is best for your health, but I can
implant good judgment with a few simple
rules. Consider these rules your sextant, compass, and map to steer clear of the rocky shoals
of an unhealthy lifestyle and toward the clear
open seas of healthy practices. Good luck and
good sailing!!

What Does a Healthy Lifestyle Include?

1 Optimal Nutrition

Follow the "Cardinal Rules" listed below.

2 Regular Exercise

A healthy lifestyle includes stretching,
strengthening, and aerobic conditioning. At the
very least, take a brisk 30 minute walk daily.
For better results, join a fitness club, get a
stair climber or cross country skiing device, or
simply follow any of the dozens of workout vid-
eos available at your local video store. Of

course, see your doctor before beginning any exercise program.

3 Toxin Avoidance

Your body is constantly working to excrete (through feces, urine, and sweat) the toxic by-products of living. In our heavily polluted industrial age, too many people are exposed to overwhelming amounts of air, water, and food pollutants that tax the body's ability to eliminate poisons.

To avoid toxins, get a water filter device for your kitchen sink. If you live in a polluted region, get politically involved to help clean up the air or move to another region. Soak fresh produce in a mild solution of warm water and ¼ c. of vinegar for 5 minutes, rinse, and then eat as usual. For more on improving your body's ability to tolerate toxins, see my book *Safe Eating*.

4 Attitude

For centuries, mystics, religious leaders, and philosophers have told us about the link between the mind and body. An abundance of research shows that the most blatant risk factor toward heart disease is loneliness. There are textbooks with thousands of scientific references showing the important link between mind and the major killers and cripplers in Western society—heart disease, cancer, diabetes, allergies, osteoporosis, mental illness, infections, and so on.

Scientists have found that our immune factors; which are "tiny soldiers" patrolling the body to destroy invading bacteria, virus, or cancer cells, have receptors for brain chemicals (neurochemical transmitters). Think about that! Each of our vital protective soldiers has a "nervous system" of sorts. When you are depressed, so is your immune system. Think love, joy, beauty, and forgiveness. Find something that you would do for free and figure out a way to be paid for it. Have someone to love, something to do, and something to look forward to. In other words, . . . *whatever is honorable, whatever is right, whatever is pure, whatever is lovely, whatever is of good repute, if there is any excellence and if anything worthy of praise, let your mind dwell on these things.* (Philippians 4:19).

5 Body Maintenance

Here are some sound tips for body maintenance. Wear comfortable shoes with good arch support, wide toes, and leather that breathes. Use a mattress that provides support without being too hard. Adjustable inflatable air mattresses are wonderful. Use a small pillow in the small part (lumbar) of your back when you sit for extended periods. Whenever possible, lie on the floor with the lower part of your legs up on a footstool to improve leg circulation. Wear a hat and use sunglasses and sunscreen lotion when in the sun. Use foam ear protectors when around loud noises. Many of these recommendations may seem obvious, but too many people expect this mortal body to withstand endless abuse and neglect. With care, your body is built to last 8 or 10 decades with dependable service.

Cardinal Rules of Nutrition

- Eat foods in or as close to their natural state as possible. Biochemists discover something new everyday to support this statement. Think of the "Divine design" that went into creating our food supply. For minimally processed foods, shop the perimeter of the grocery store.

- Eat a wide variety of foods. While there are some very nutrient-dense foods that should be included often in your diet, there are no perfect foods that have all the essential nutrients. By eating a variety of plant and animal foods, you are much more likely to include essential, but poorly-understood, nutrients.

- Eat small frequent meals, relying more on 4-6 small snacks per day rather than 1-3 huge meals.
- Minimize intake of fat, salt, sugar, cholesterol, alcohol, and caffeine. Avoid processed meats (luncheon, smoked, and salted meats) and food additives, especially nitrites, MSG, and food colorings.
- Maximize intake of fresh vegetables, fruit, whole grains, beans, fish, poultry, lowfat dairy products, and clean water. These should constitute the staples of your diet. Mentally cut up your dinner plate into pie sections where ⅔ is unprocessed plant food and ⅓ is lowfat, high-protein animal food. This is the ancestral diet for most humans.
- For people who eat meat, select animals that fly, swim, or run. Cows are locked in stationary positions to build fat and weight. Minimize beef intake.

Finally, as an overall test of your food use this.

> ***If it will not sprout or rot, don't eat it!***
>
> If a food cannot nourish a bacteria cell,
> it cannot nourish your body cells.

Getting Your Nutrients

Get your nutrients with a fork and spoon—
through food. Realistically, due to stress, pol-
lution, sedentary lives, and junk food, we cannot obtain optimal amounts of nutrients
through food alone. Hence, a quality broad
spectrum vitamin-mineral supplement is valuable for all people and essential for most people. The following is a list of nutrients that
should be taken regularly to help reduce the
incidence and severity of disease, delay the
aging process, and improve vitality, fertility,
and awareness. You can find a broad spectrum
vitamin available from several vendors listed
in the Appendix or at your health food store.

Nutrient

Supplemental Range

Vitamins

A (beta-carotene) _____ 10,000-25,000 iu
D (cholecalciferol)_____400-800 iu
E (mixed natural tocopherols)_____800-2400 iu
K (phytonadione) _____100-1000 mcg
B-1 (thiamin)_____ 4-50 mg
B-2 (riboflavin) _____ 4-50 mg
B-3 (niacinamide)_____20-200 mg
B-6 (pyridoxine) _____ 6-50 mg
B-12 (cobalamin)_____12-1000 mcg
folacin (folic acid) _____400-800 mcg
biotin (biotin)_____300-600 mcg
C (ascorbic acid) _____500-5000 mg
pantothenic acid _____30-100 mg
choline (as bitartrate) _____250-500 mg

Minerals

calcium (ionized, or citrate) _____400-800 mg
magnesium (ionized, or citrate) _____400-800 mg
zinc (picolinate)_____ 15-50 mg
iron (chelated) _____ 10-30 mg
copper (chelated)_____ 1-3 mg
iodine (potassium iodide) _____150-1000 mcg
manganese (chelated) _____ 5-10 mg
chromium (picolinate, or yeast)_____200-400 mcg
molybdenum (chelated)_____150-300 mcg
selenium (selenomethionine)_____200-400 mcg
silicon (Mg-trisilicate) _____ 10-20 mg
vanadium (Na-metavanadate)_____ 10-20 mcg
EPA (fish oil) _____ 1-2 T., or 3-6 caps

Appendix C—References

Primary Textbooks
and Excellent General Reading

Carper, J., *The Food Pharmacy,*
(NY: Bantam Books, 1988).

Gottlieb, W. (ed.), *Doctors Book of Home Remedies,* (Emmaus, PA: Rodale Press, 1990).

Hausman, P., and JB Hurley, *Healing Foods,*
(NY: Dell, 1989).

Jarvis, DC, *Folk Medicine*, (NY: Fawcett Crest, 1958)

Kaptchuk, T., and Croucher, M., *The Healing Arts,*
(NY: Summit Books, 1987).

Kerr, RW, *Herbalism Through the Ages,*
(Kingsport, TN: Kingsport Press, 1969).

Langer, SE, *Solved: The Riddle of Illness,*
(New Canaan, CT: Keats, 1984).

Lau, BL, *Garlic for Health,*
(Wilmot, WI: Lotus Light, 1988).

Lieberman, S., and Bruning, N., *The Real Vitamin and Mineral Book,* (NY: Avery, 1990).

Lucas, R., *Secrets of the Chinese Herbalists,*
(W. Nyack, NY: Parker Publ, 1977).

Lust, J., *The Herb Book,* (NY: Bantam Books, 1974).

McGrath, W., *Amish Folk Remedies,*
(Freeport Press, 1985).

Meyer, C., *American Folk Medicine,*
(Glenwood, IL: Meyerbooks, 1985).

Mowrey, DB, *Scientific Validation of Herbal Medicine,*
(New Canaan, CT: Keats, 1986).

Murray, MT, *Healing Power of Herbs,*
(Sacramento: Prima, 1991).

Murray, MT, and Pizzorno, J., *Encyclopedia of Natural Medicine,* (Sacramento: Prima, 1990).

Quillin, P, *Healing Nutrients,* (NY: Random House, 1987).

Rinzler, CA, *Feed a Cold, Starve a Fever,* (NY: Facts on File, 1991).

Royal, PC, *Herbally Yours,* (Hurricane, UT: Sound Nutrition, 1982).

Tierra, M, *The Way of Herbs,* (NY: Pocket Books, 1990).

Weaver, SM, *Grandma's Home Remedies,* (Millersburg, OH: Fani's Books, 1988).

Weiner, M., *Weiner's Herbal,* (Mill Valley, CA: Quantum Books, 1990).

Werbach, M., *Nutritional Influences on Illness,* (Tarzana, CA: Third Line Press, 1993).

Selected Scientific References
Referred to Within the Text

[1]Quillin, P., *Healing Nutrients*. (New York: Random House, 1987).

[2]Random House Encyclopedia (New York: Random House, 1983), 745.

[3]Murray, MT, *Healing Power of Herbs*, (Sacramento: Prima Publ., 1991) 1.

[4]*The Complete Drug Reference*, (Yonkers, NY: Consumers Union, 1992), 372.

[5]Duke, JA, *Handbook of Medicinal Herbs,* (Boca Raton, FL: CRC Press, 1985). See also Leung, AY, *Encyclopedia of Common Natural Ingredients Used in Food, Drugs, and Cosmetics,* (NY: John Wiley Press, 1980).

[6]Nassar, BA, et al., *Nutrition Research*, 1986. vol. 6:1397.

[7]Downing, DT, et al., *Journal of American Academy of Dermatology,* 1980. vol. 14:221.

[8]Schachner, L., *Pediatric Clinics of North America,* 1980. vol. 30:337.

[9]Cunliffe, J., *British Journal of Dermatology,* 1981.
vol. 117:160.

[10]Verna, KC, et al., *Acta Dermatovener,* 1980.
vol. 60:337.

[11]Elias, PM, et al., *Archives of Dermatology,* 1981.
vol. 20:278.

[12]McCarty, M., *Medical Hypotheses,* 1984. vol. 14:307.

[13]Michaelsson, G., et al., *Acta Dermto-Venerologica,* 1984.
vol. 64:9.

[14]Hendler, SS, *The Doctors' Vitamin and Mineral Encyclopedia,* (NY: Simon & Schuster, 1990)
See also Davies, S., and A. Stewart, *Nutritional Medicine,* (NY: Avon, 1987).

[15]Werbach, MR, *Nutritional Influences on Illness* (Tarzana, CA: Third Line Press, 1992).

[16]Williams, RJ, *The Prevention of Alcoholism Through Nutrition,* (NY: Bantam, 1981).

[17]Krohn, J., *Allergy Relief and Prevention,* (Pt. Roberts, WA: Hartley & Marks, 1991).

[18]Burr, ML, et al., *Human Nutrition: Applied Nutrition,* Oct. 1985. vol. 39A:349.
See also Pelikan, Z., et al., *Annals of Allergy,* Mar. 1987. vol. 58:164.

[19]Koepke, JW, et al., *Annals of Allergy,* Mar. 1985.
vol. 54:213.

[20]Reynolds, RD, et al., *Federation Proceedings,* 1984.
vol. 43:470.

[21]Mohsenin, L., et al., *American Review of Respiratory Disease,* 1983. vol. 127:143.

[22]Okayama, H., et al., *Journal of American Medical Association,* Feb. 27, 1987. vol. 257:1076.

[23]Balch, JF, and PA Balch, *Prescription for Nutritional Healing,* (NY: Avery, 1990), 100.

[24]Murray, M., and J. Pizzorno, *Encyclopedia of Natural Medicine,* (Sacramento: Prima, 1990).

[25]Crook, WG, *Help for the Hyperactive Child,* (Jackson, TN: Professional Books, 1991).

[26]Machlin, LJ, *Handbook of Vitamins,* (NY: Marcel Dekker, 1991), 145.

[27]Hendler, SS, ibid. p. 247.

[28]Werbach, M., ibid, p. 47.

[29]Quillin, P., in Hetter (ed.), *Lipoplasty* (Boston: Little, Brown, 1990), 209.

[30]Whitaker, J., *Health and Healing,* Jan. 1993. vol. 3 no. 1:4.

[31]Werbach, M., ibid. p. 196.

[32]Hendler, SS, ibid. p. 87.

[33]Eby, GA, et al., *Antimicrobial Agents and Chemotherapy,* 1984. vol. 25:20.

[34]Lewin, S., *Vitamin C: Its Molecular Biology and Medical Potential,* (NY: Van Nostrand Reinhold, 1974).

[35]Terezhalmy, GT, et al., *Oral Surgery,* 1978. vol. 45:56.

[36]Starasoler, S., et al., *NY State Dental Journal,* 1978. vol. 44 no. 9:382.

[37]Griffith, RS, *Dermatologica,* 1987. vol. 175:183

[38]Quillin, P., ibid, p. 344.

[39]Quillin, P., ibid, p. 294.

[40]Budoff, PW, *No More Hot Flashes,* (NY: Warner, 1983)

[41]Werbach, MR, ibid, p. 376.

[42]Johnson, ES, et al., *British Medical Journal,* Aug. 1985. vol. 291:569.

[43]Quillin, P., ibid, p. 81.

[44]Leathwood, P., et al., *Pharmacological Biochemistry Behavior,* 1982. vol. 17:65.
See also Leathwood, P., et al., *Planta Medica,* 1985. vol. 54:144.

[45]Prodromos, PN, et al., *Southwest Medicine,* 1968.
vol 47:17.
See also Sternliev, P., *New England Journal of Medicine,* 1963. vol. 268:57.

[46]Vorberg, G., *Clinical Trials Journal,* 1985. vol. 22:149.

[47]Mowrey, D., et al. *Lancet,* 1982. vol. i:665.

[48]Champlault, G., et al., *British Journal of Clinical Pharmacology,* 1984. vol. 18:461.

[49]Langer, SE, *Solved: The Riddle of Illness,* (New Canaan, CT: Keats, 1984), 40.

Other books you'll want--

Cooking with the Horse and Buggy People

Discover over 600 Amish recipes by Amish ladies from Holmes and Wayne counties—the heart of Ohio's Amish Country. Learn Amish secrets for breads, cakes, cookies desserts, pies, salads, main dishes, soups, cereals, candy, drinks, canning tips, preparing wild game and others.   ($12.95 plus $2.00 s. & h. 2/$20.00 total)

To order: Print your name and address and the words *Amish Cooking* on a piece of paper and mail it along with a check or money order to: The Leader Co., Inc. Publishing Division, Dept. CH101, 931 North Main Street, North Canton, OH 44720. Include card number and expiration date to order by MasterCard or Visa.

- **Cleanse Your Arteries & Save Your Life.** Learn doctors' tips on chest pain and clogged arteries and other health tips, such as the dangers in health food products and cholesterol-reduction diets.
- **How to Protect Your Financial Security.** Protect your life savings from a defect in Medicare.

    Important reading for every senior citizen considering nursing home care.

- **Little Known Health Cures.** Find out what can enhance alertness and may improve memory. Learn what nutrients scientists say may slow down aging and other health cures doctors don't usually share.
- **How to Turn Your Trash into Cash.** One person's trash is another's $35,000 treasure. Read this book before you throw out anything.

Write The Leader Company for prices and ordering information.

Also by Dr. Patrick Quillan

Beating Cancer with Nutrition

Educates about cancer, current therapies, and the devastating effects of treatment. Examines the laws of nutrition and the link to cancer. Shows how nutrients can prevent hair loss, mouth sores, and organ damage from chemotherapy.

Describes malnutrition in the cancer patient, and how the program strategy helps to

enhance the body's tunor-killing capacity and bolster the immune system.

Buy it, or additional copies of *Amish Folk Medicine,* at your bookstore, or call toll-free, day or night,

800/444-2524